12 Secrets to Virility

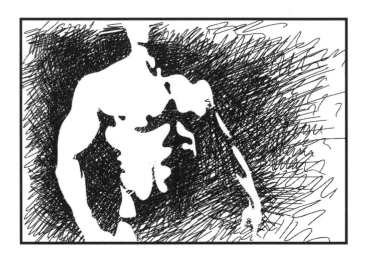

A Man's Guide to Peak Health, Great Sex and Powerful Living

D0757290

Al Sears, MD

Warning-Disclaimer: Dr. Al Sears wrote this book to provide information in regard to the subject matter covered. It is offered with the understanding that the publisher and the author are not liable for the misconception or misuse of the information provided.

Every effort has been made to make this book as complete and accurate as possible. The purpose of this book is to educate. The author and the publisher shall have neither liability nor responsibility to any person or entity with respect to any loss, damage, or injury caused or alleged to be caused directly or indirectly by the information contained in this book.

The information presented herein is in no way intended as a substitute for medical counseling or medical attention.

Published by:
Al Sears, MD
12794 W. Forest Hill Blvd.
Suite 16
Wellington, FL 33414

http://www.alsearsmd.com

$39.90

This book is dedicated to my brother Dave... for being Dave.

Meet Dr. Sears

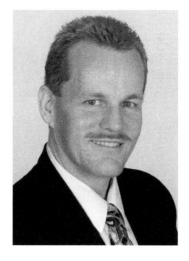

Dr. Al Sears is fast becoming the nation's leading authority on longevity and heart health. Since the release of his latest book, *The Doctor's Heart Cure*, he has been interviewed on over two dozen nationally syndicated radio programs with an audience of millions.

In just three years, Dr. Sears has published over 325 articles and 3 books in the fields of alternative medicine, anti-aging and nutritional supplementation - including a monthly subscription newsletter entitled *Health Confidential for Men*.

His cutting edge breakthroughs and commanding knowledge of alternative medicine have been transforming the lives of his patients for over 15 years.

Dr. Sears currently owns and operates a successful integrative medicine and anti-aging clinic in Wellington, Florida with over 15,000 patients. Over the course of his career, he has developed his own approach to heart health, longevity and anti-aging medicine - combining the best of modern medical science with natural holistic techniques and treatments.

He is a member of the American Academy of Anti-Aging Medicine, a diplomat of the American Board of Anti-Aging Medicine and is Board Certified in Anti-Aging Medicine. He is an avid researcher and enthusiastic lecturer in this exciting new field of medicine.

In 2002, he was appointed to the international panel of experts at Health Sciences Institute, (HSI) a worldwide consulting service for integrative healthcare. He is also an adjunct professor at Barry University where he teaches courses in human anatomy, physiology and nutrition. As well as being a lifelong advocate of nutritional supplementation and exercise programs, Dr. Sears is an ACE certified fitness trainer.

Dr. Sears is the founder and director of The Wellness Research Foundation, which is conducting original research to evaluate natural alternatives to pharmaceutical therapies.

His practice houses "The McCormick-Green Center for Integrative Therapies", a nonprofit charity devoted to research and the education of the public and other physicians. Also maintained at his practice, is an herbal apothecary of over 250 organic herbs used for research, education and treatments.

Introduction

Dear Reader,

Congratulations on taking an important step toward restoring your virility!

I am confident that you will find it to be a good choice. In fact, I don't know of anywhere else you could turn for a solution to this problem – the problem of keeping your best masculine features in our modern environment.

Don't get me wrong... We have so many advances to be thankful for in our modern world ... I'm not suggesting that you give them up.

Yet recognizing that some of these advances have come at the price of previous environmental benefits is the first step to putting together the best of both worlds – combining our modern medical and technological achievements with the advantages of our harsh and primitive, yet pristine environment.

The undeniable fact is that you find yourself living in a world dramatically different form the one that selected our physical and chemical adaptations. From just a few thousand years ago, back through the millions of years of human existence our world was relatively constant. This means that for over 99.9% of our human ascent to such spectacular planetary dominance the rules of survival were the same.

Now, like a 747 turning on a dime, we've changed our interaction with our world. Your physical activity is totally different. Not only do we no longer hunt for our food, but your food has been dramatically altered and continues to be altered further (mostly without your knowledge or consent). In an evolutionary blink of an eye, we removed ourselves from the world we were built for and created a new one.

This mismatch between our genetic adaptations and our modern environment is the cause of the greatest epidemic in the history of humankind –maturity onset heart disease. This view of the cause points to an obvious strategy for the cure. It is the basis for my previous book, *The Doctor's Heart Cure*.

Yet this irony of the pinnacle of adaptive perfection overwhelmed by the degree and pace of its changes to its own living conditions is even more apparent when it comes to the sexual health of the American male.

> ➤ Sperm counts are going down in America and most of the rest of the Western World.
> ➤ Erectile dysfunction has become the accepted norm for middle aged men.
> ➤ Pharmaceutical companies make billions from this market, which hardly existed just 15 years ago.
> ➤ About 10% of the older men coming to my clinic have more female estrogen than male testosterone.
> ➤ Waist lines and prostates continue to grow while penises and libidos shrink.

Do you need more evidence that these changes are coming from the environment? Well, both the mighty Florida panther and the extremely evolutionarily stable alligator have shrinking penises documented over just a couple of generations living in the Everglades near sewage sites!

Yes, our ancestors had it tough. But they never had their very manhood threatened in this way. You have a new challenge. As a man today, you need to understand how these changes are sapping your strength, taking your energy and in many cases turning you into a woman.

Become aware of this threat and take action to avert the consequences!

Specializing in anti-aging medicine, sexual health and fitness in over 15,000 patients, I've seen thousands of men come into my office suffering from the effects of their modern environment with:

- Fatigue and Depression
- Low Sex Drive
- Physical Weakness
- Excess Fat and Obesity
- Swollen Prostate
- Flagging Mental Capacity
- Muscle and Joint Pain

Once these men realize the cause, it's apparent that change is possible. A whole new world opens up to them. Instead of feeling like helpless victims, they can take action to restore the natural power of real manhood. Many tell me that this is what they were always looking for – but were never able to express in words.

Over the years, several of my patients asked me to put these techniques together in writing. To better understand the secrets of male vitality, I have grouped the most important insights into twelve core ideas – the *12 Secrets to Virility.*

Each chapter is a wake-up call to the powers lying dormant in your own body. And each provides practical advice you can immediately apply to your own life.

You can use each chapter as a stand-alone guide but I suggest that you start with the first secret, testosterone. It is the most fundamental element in most men's virility. It's the foundation of manhood – and the substance most under threat by today's environment.

In addition, many of the toxins in your environment have a chemical structure that closely resembles estrogen. These "estrogen mimics" travel through your body and attach themselves to estrogen receptors in your organs and tissues.

As fake estrogens, they send out instructions that start to break down and feminize your body. As the years go by, your sex drive begins to disappear, your belly and face become bloated and your drive and ambition start to fade. From there, other problems begin to develop – slowly pushing you towards lethargy and disease.

This problem with estrogens from your environment is the second secret and also one you don't want to skip.

Each secret in this book is written to specifically address each aspect of male health and sexual vitality. In each chapter, you'll find practical and easy-to-follow strategies designed to reconnect you to the energy and power you were born to control.

By the time you finish the final secret, you'll be armed with the ammunition you need to reclaim your power as a man.

If you follow these simple steps in this book, you will…

• Radiate confidence and take control of every situation – whether it's charming the ladies or confronting challenges in your career.

• Regain the strength and muscle mass of your younger days. Watch as your fat melts away to reveal well-defined muscle and a masculine taper.

• Have spontaneous and rock-hard erections. Imagine your excitement when you realize that all night sex isn't just for college kids.

• Boost your brainpower – and your memory. You'll develop a focus and clarity of mind that will generate new ideas and solve problems at lightning speed.

• Live with both strength and mobility. Experience the privilege of getting older without disabling aging. You'll be playing golf and traveling the world while your peers are stuck in wheelchairs and retirement homes.

As you read this special report, let go of the limitations that hold you back from being the kind of man you know you can be. Open yourself to the promise of great strength and passion. You've had the potential all along.

Now use the *12 Secrets to Virility* to help you unlock it.

To Your Good Health,
Al Sears, MD

PS. If you haven't done so yet you can contact me at www.AlSearsMD.com. You can sign up for my Health Confidential Newsletter and get free updates to this book.

Table of Contents

Secret #1

Ride with the King: Testosterone

Testosterone... A Man's Best Advantage

Testosterone is man's primary masculine hormone. It's what makes you strong, smart, quick and aggressive. It's what makes you a potent and virile lover. It's what gives you the drive to succeed... to win at sports, profit at business, shock the world with your art and romance the ladies with your poetry.

Testosterone is what makes you feel invulnerable in your twenties and thirties. And the reduction of testosterone in your body is what makes you feel weaker, slower and more breakable as you age.

Science shows that by getting his body to produce youthful levels of testosterone, an older man can enjoy the following benefits:

- A Thin, Lean Abdomen

- Spontaneous Erections

- Impressive Muscularity

- Remarkable Stamina

- Mental Alertness

- A Stronger Heart

- An Iron-Clad Immune System

- And Much More…

Testosterone Defines Manhood

Most of the qualities we think of when we consider the manly virtues – bravery, assertiveness, certitude and valor – are present when the body is flushed with testosterone.

An essay in *The New York Times Magazine* points out that:

- Bosses have more testosterone than their workers.

- Trial lawyers have more than tax lawyers.

- Commodity traders have higher levels than the back office crew.

- Actors have more than ministers.

And it's true for women, too. Working women have higher testosterone levels than stay at home moms.

The message from nature is crystal clear:

The One with the Most Testosterone Wins

You can tell who won a tennis match without knowing the final score… just sample their T levels throughout the match. In this example, "love" equals low testosterone.

It's even true for people watching a game. A 1998 study found that fans backing the winning side in a college basketball game saw their T levels rise. Fans rooting for the losers saw theirs fall.

Matt Ridley, in his book "The Red Queen" says, "If you lose a contest with prey or a rival, it makes sense not to pick another fight immediately. So your body wisely prompts you to withdraw, filling your brain with depression and self-doubt."

One of my colleagues, Karlis Ullis, a medical director at UCLA and an internationally recognized authority on men's health, puts it this way:

"Testosterone is a near magic substance that makes a man a man! There is no other substance on the planet, natural or man made, that can have such profound affects. It can restore or boost sex drive in men of virtually any age. It can decrease fat tissue and increase muscle tissue. It can sharpen the mind and build confidence. It can increase overall energy levels and boost mental acuity."

Testosterone Lowers Your Risk of Chronic Disease

Testosterone does more than make you manly. It also protects you from a long list of diseases:

- Heart Disease

- Stroke

- Alzheimer's

- Osteoporosis

- Type II Diabetes

- Depression

- Obesity

It's not surprising that these illnesses are most common in men over forty.   Much of "natural aging process" is all about the loss of testosterone.

The Gods Are Fickle... What They Give, They Also Take Away

When you're in your twenties and early thirties, you have all the testosterone you need. As a result, you have energy, grit and clear ideas.

But testosterone declines with age. As testosterone declines, so do your mental and physical abilities. It starts in your early thirties and, little by little, gets worse every day. By the time you're in your mid forties, there are real signs of decline, in your anatomy and in your functional capacity.

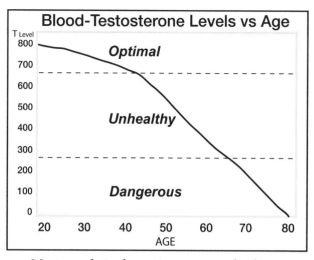

Most people in the mainstream medical community accept this degradation as inevitable. What the body does "naturally," let the body do, they say.

For you, as a mature man, this is the equivalent of saying, "Crawl up in a corner and die."

I don't believe you have to accept such an unhappy fate. I believe – in fact, I know – that you can slow down and even reverse much of the debilitation that comes from aging.

I know you can because I've seen positive results from countless patients I've worked with. I've seen the results in my brother. *I've experienced the results myself.*

You can prevent the cruel effects of aging... and you can do so naturally and safely by keeping your natural testosterone production high.

The Story of Joe: Slower, Fatter and Smaller

Joe, a 48-year-old mechanic came to my clinic in south Florida from the West Coast. He had read my book on natural testosterone boosting.

"You gotta help me doctor," he said. "You're my last hope."

My nurse wrote on his chart, "Erectile dysfunction for twenty years." Erectile dysfunction or ED, is the politically correct way to say "impotence."

Further down on the chart it read, "Also complaining of weight gain, fatigue, general weakness, lack of motivation, memory loss and depression."

Joe was the walking personification of testosterone deficiency: The sad drooping eyes. The defeated expression. The forward slumped shoulders and potbelly. The soft, "dough-boy" look. A single defined muscle was nowhere in sight. Just rolls of hanging flab.

He had seen other doctors before me. "They gave me Viagra, but it didn't do anything. Everyone said Viagra was supposed to be so great. Do you have any idea why Viagra didn't work for me, Doctor."

"Yes," I said. "Because you're not suffering from a deficiency of Viagra."

Low Testosterone Causes More than Just Impotence

I told Joe that much of what he was experiencing was caused by a deficiency of testosterone. Specifically, his fatigue, abdominal weight gain, decreased sex drive and erectile dysfunction.

"You may have noticed something else…" I advised him. "Your penis may seem smaller."

"It does." Joe admitted.

Joe isn't alone. Most American men – and men from other modern, industrialized countries – suffer from dangerously low levels of testosterone. And because of the rise of environmental toxins, things are getting worse.

In my twenty-five years of clinical experience with men's health, I've seen the trend worsen. It's getting tougher for an aging man to stay manly… and that's an unnecessary shame.

As a man ages, his testosterone decreases while his estrogen increases. This is partly due to a conversion of testosterone to estrogen. One study I know of found that estrogen levels in an average 54-year-old man are higher than those in an average 59-year-old woman.

As shocking as it sounds, you may have more estrogen than a woman.

And the problem compounds itself. Lower levels of testosterone makes it more likely that you'll be fat. And when you have a potbelly, it tends to accelerate the negative testosterone/estrogen (T/ E) imbalance.

Studies show that fat cells, especially gut fat, generate the aromatase enzyme that converts testosterone to estrogen. That's why I'm never surprised when a pot-bellied patient measures "very low" on the testosterone meter and "too high" for estrogen.

It's a vicious cycle of decreasing testosterone and increasing estrogen. You start to look and feel more like a woman but your mind, and your culture, still expect you to be a man!

And it's not just how you look and feel. When a man's T/E ratio declines it also increases the risk of heart attack and stroke. And high levels of estrogen in men are implicated in benign prostatic hypertrophy (BPH). That's the enlargement of the prostate gland at the base of the penis that makes it difficult to begin urinating...and even harder to stop.

The Danger of the Low-Fat Diet

In addition to all the artificial toxins we're exposed to, some well-intentioned medical "help" is lowering our testosterone even further.

The most common form of medical malpractice is recommending the low fat (read high carb) diet. Since most doctors know little to nothing about nutrition, it only makes sense that they often recommend the diet endorsed by mainstream medical organizations such as the American Medical Association, (AMA) and the American Heart Association, (AHA).

These low fat diets are actually high carb killers. In seeking to cut out "fatty" meats and cholesterol, they substitute man-made poisons such as pastas and breads and tubers.

I will cover this subject in detail later in the book. For the moment let me point out that there are, literally, hundreds of studies that demonstrate the dangers of high-carb, low-fat diets. A powerful example is a recent Swedish study. They found that, "switching from a high to a low fat diet *lowered blood testosterone levels by 10 percent.*"[1]

Here's the bottom line: to be healthy in a manly way – slim, strong, virile and energetic – you need a healthy balance of high testosterone and low estrogen. To get that, you need to do two things:

1. Avoid Unnatural Contaminants that Artificially Lower Your Testosterone and Increase Estrogen, and...

2. Boost Your Testosterone Naturally.

Before we go any further, let's see where you stand in terms of testosterone/estrogen balance. Take a few minutes to answer a few questions about yourself and see how you score.

The Dr Sears "20 Questions" Testosterone Test

	1. Frequently	2. Occasionally	3. Never
1. Do you have trouble obtaining an erection?	___	___	___
2. Do you lose your erection before orgasm?	___	___	___
3. When attempting sexual intercourse, how often is it unsatisfactory for you?	___	___	___
4. Have you noticed a decreased desire for sex?	___	___	___
5. Does your partner want sex more than you?	___	___	___
6. Do you smoke tobacco?	___	___	___
7. Do you struggle with a lack of ambition and motivation?	___	___	___
8. Do you lack the energy to perform your daily chores?	___	___	___
9. Do you become moody, depressed or irritable without good reason?	___	___	___
10. Do you lack the strength to lift heavy household objects?	___	___	___
11. Do you lack the desire to get up in the morning?	___	___	___
12. Are you disinterested in exercising?	___	___	___

(Continued on the next page...)

	1. Frequently	2. Occasionally	3. Never
13. Do you use less weight at the gym?	_____	_____	_____
14. Do you skip exercise sessions?	_____	_____	_____
15. How often do you need a caffeine boost?	_____	_____	_____
16. How often do you unintentionally fall asleep when you sit down after dinner?	_____	_____	_____
17. Do you deny yourself food to keep from gaining weight?	_____	_____	_____
18. How many prescription drugs do you regularly take?	3 or more	1-2	None
19. Pinch your fat just to the side of your belly button; how much can you pinch?:	> 1"	about 1"	< 1"
20. What is your age?	> 50	35-50	< 35

SCORING:

Score 10 points for each response in column 3
     5 points for each response in column 2
     0 points for each response in column 1

Total: _____

Interpretation:

Above 150:   You're a **STUD!** Keep up the good work.

120 – 150:   **AVERAGE.** You may be one of the many men suffering from falling testosterone levels.

Below 120:   **DEFICIENT.** You would likely benefit from natural testosterone boosting.

Below 100:   **SUFFERING.** You need immediate help from boosting testosterone.

How did you score?

If you scored above 150, chances are you are either very fortunate or very young. If you scored below 120, try my testosterone boosting program and take the test again in about 6 weeks.

Get All the Benefits... But Do It Right

If you scored poorly on the test above you probably need to improve your testosterone profile. You can – and should – do it naturally.

But to be sure, get your testosterone measured by your doctor. On your lab report, you will see a "normal range" for testosterone. It's usually from about 250 to 850 ng/dl.

But here's the rub. Many men in my practice who have testosterone levels in the lower third of the "normal" range, will have the symptoms of testosterone deficiency described above. When I boost their testosterone levels to the upper one third of the normal range these symptoms quickly resolve.

It is very important for men to have their estrogen levels measured, too. But your doctor probably won't measure it unless you ask. Estrogen levels for men are the opposite of testosterone. You want you estrogen to be lower than average. We shoot for a level below 100 pc/ml.

Once you have the results from your physical and blood work, you can start turning yourself into the man you were meant to be.

Boost Your Testosterone... *Naturally*

Many men over 40 feel drained. Their sex drive isn't what it used to be, they don't have the energy they used to have, they feel depressed, and often weaker than they used to.

When you're testosterone levels begin to fall, the ratio between estrogen and testosterone increases. You also acquire excess estrogens through your environment—pollutants, many foods, and even the water you drink can contain estrogen or estrogen-like compounds. The estrogen that bombards your body from outside sources further contributes to imbalanced hormone levels. And these higher relative levels of estrogen cause health problems.

Normally, your testosterone level is ten times higher than your estrogen level. But with falling testosterone levels and rising estrogen levels, the balance of these two hormones gets all out of whack.

High estrogen levels in a man can swell the prostate. It can cause your muscles to weaken and atrophy. It leads to weight gain, especially fat. It contributes to moodiness. And it attacks you sex drive.

Fortunately, you can do many things to boost your testosterone and to control rising estrogen levels – all of them safe and natural. In the following pages I'll tell you about a number of natural supplements that help boost your testosterone, keep your sex drive running strong, and bring your estrogen levels under control.

I'll give you specific recommendations for how much of each supplement you should take—or how you can find out what the optimum dose is for you.

First, let's take a look at the best ways to control estrogen. With the right supplements, your body can metabolize estrogen naturally, helping to restore the testosterone/estrogen balance.

The two supplements that work best are DIM and Indole-3-Carbinol.

DIM

DIM is short for diindolylmethane. It's a naturally occurring plant compound, found commonly in cruciferous vegetables. Things like broccoli, cauliflower, asparagus, Brussels sprouts, and cabbage contain high levels of DIM. DIM helps the body to metabolize estrogen. It works to break down estrogen into safer compounds, clearing away the potential damaging hormone.

One study conducted in the Department of Molecular and Cell Biology at UC Berkeley examined the urine of patients taking DIM versus those not taking the supplement. The count of estrogen metabolites in the urine of those taking DIM was significantly higher than the control group. In other words, this study shows that DIM helps the body to break down estrogen.[2]

Indole-3-Carbinol

Indole-3-carbinol is another compound found in cruciferous vegetables, and is actually the precursor to DIM. I prefer DIM, if I have to choose between the two, but they're both good, and they work well in combination. One of the most dangerous effects of excess estrogen is an increase in certain cancer risks. Estrogen contributes to the growth of tumors, especially in sex glands and organs. Indole-3-carbinol protects cells from cancer and mutation, properties that show a lot of promise in dealing with excess estrogen and its dangers.[3] Researchers at the Department of Microbiology at New York Medical College have closely examined the mechanism of Indole-3-carbinol and found that it interferes with the body's receptors for certain types of estradiols. It also helps to form compounds that metabolize estrogen.[4]

Recommended Dosages: For men I recommend taking 200 to 400 mg of DIM each day and that you take 200mg of Indole-3-Carbinol each day. Or you can eat a pound of cruciferous vegetables, but I find most of patients object to that suggestion.

The Ban on Being a Man

Bringing the ratio of estrogen and testosterone into balance is immensely beneficial to your health, but for most men, that alone isn't enough. You also need to boost your testosterone levels back up to normal, back into the range where you feel good...virile.

My favorite method of naturally boosting testosterone is to use supplements from the "andro" family. Andro supplements are naturally occurring hormones that act as precursors to testosterone production in the body. Even low levels of androstenedione can markedly boost your levels of testosterone. One study showed low doses increased testosterone levels on average by as much as 183%.[5]

Unfortunately, in April 2004, androstenedione became illegal. The FDA banned it, and not for very good reasons either. I was disappointed to find one of the safest ways to boost men's health no longer available without a prescription.

Fortunately, there are alternatives to andros that are quite effective in their own right.

DHEA

The testosterone precursor that I now recommend for best results is DHEA. Its scientific name is dehyroepiandrosterone, but that's such a mouthful. DHEA is a perfectly legal and perfectly safe substance for naturally boosting your body's testosterone output.

Your body produces DHEA naturally. Your adrenal glands secrete DHEA into your system where it's converted into testosterone and other useful substances. DHEA is the most abundant hormone in your body, but as you get older, your levels of DHEA begin to decline. By the time you're 65, your body produces just 10% of the DHEA that it produced when you were 20.

DHEA provides many benefits in addition to boosting your body's own natural testosterone. It's linked to bone health, proper insulin balance, a sense of well-being, weight loss, an improved libido, and healthier connective tissues.[6]

One of the reasons DHEA is so important is that it helps to lower your cortisol levels. Cortisol is a product of stress. Remember, one of the most damaging things to your health—and to your sex life—is stress. Now, in a life-or-death situation, cortisol is great. It directs all of your body's resources to survival—you can run faster, lift heavy objects, fight like a lion… but if you're not facing a life-or-death situation, cortisol wreaks havoc on the body. It directs all your resources away from maintenance and repair. And that accelerates aging.

Most of my stressed out patients are _chronically_ stressed. As a result, they have chronically high levels of cortisol. That means their DHEA levels are usually below where they should be. And low DHEA usually means low testosterone.

It means other things, too. People with low levels of DHEA generally don't live as long. They get sick more often, are more susceptible to inflammatory diseases (inflammation has recently been linked to heart disease and damaged arteries, so they are at higher risk for these conditions, too), they are depressed more often, they don't think as clearly, and they don't look as good.

On the other hand, people with higher levels of DHEA perform better in physical and cognitive tests.

They also:

• Experience lower stress levels.

• Enjoy more energy.

• Spend less time being sick.

• Are slimmer and trimmer.

• Enjoy more sex.

• Retain their memories better.

• Look healthy and more youthful.

Medical research has done a lot to document the health benefits of DHEA supplementation:

• The Institute of Biomedical Research at the University of Birmingham in England studied patients with poorly functioning adrenal glands.

DHEA supplementation improved their sex steroid levels. This led to improvements in well-being, energy levels, mood, and libido. The authors of this study note the importance of establishing a DHEA deficiency or an androgen deficiency before beginning supplementation.[7]

• Russian researchers set out to find the relationship between DHEA levels, erectile dysfunction, and libido in patients with chronic prostatitis. They found that patients with low DHEA levels were more likely to have erectile dysfunction. Men with higher levels of DHEA in their blood stream, tended to have the most success with achieving and maintaining an erection.[8] Austrian researchers from the University of Vienna conducted a double blind, placebo-controlled study on the relationship between healthy DHEA levels and the ability to achieve and maintain a healthy erection. Though the study was small, the results confirm that DHEA supplementation is a helpful treatment for erectile dysfunction.[9]

• In a placebo-controlled, randomized, double-blind study, researchers from the Washington School of Medicine showed that DHEA supplementation helps to prevent abdominal obesity and may be a useful treatment in metabolic syndrome. (Metabolic syndrome is a condition where six or more risk factors for heart disease and diabetes are present.) Researchers in this study administered 50 mg of DHEA to the trial group over the course of six months. The DHEA-treated patients saw significant decreases in visceral fat, subcutaneous fat, and insulin levels. They also saw a significant increase in insulin sensitivity.[10] By offering protection against insulin resistance and reducing fat levels, DHEA provides a significant overall health benefit. Indirectly, reducing fat and improving your body's use of insulin can have a number of other benefits, including higher levels of energy, a better feeling about yourself, and lowered risk of cardiovascular diseases.

• Researchers from the University of Cambridge conducted a review of studies on DHEA and a personal sense of well-being. They analyzed and cross-checked the results of the studies that met their criteria and found that 67% of men taking DHEA felt that their sense of well-being improved significantly.[11]

Aging, declining virility, waning libido—they are all caused by the decline of important hormones. It's a problem that needs to be treated holistically. DHEA is a great part of a holistic approach—it helps you to control stress, it boosts your natural testosterone production, and it can improve your mood overall.

DHEA supplementation is simple and effective. But like any hormone, too much can be just as bad as too little. Have your DHEA levels checked by a doctor before you begin supplementing. A simple blood test is all you need. Youthful DHEA levels for men fall between 300 and 500 mg/dl.

If you and your doctor discover your levels are low, discuss the best supplemental dosage based on your current DHEA levels and the optimum level you want to reach.

The bottom line is that if you have low testosterone or low DHEA levels, then DHEA supplementation is a good place to start. It will make you feel better, it will make you look better, and it will help to restore your virility and youth.

Recommendation: Work with your doctor to determine the best dosage for you based upon your current hormone levels and your optimum hormone levels. For most of my patient's with low DHEA levels, I have them begin with a 10 mg daily dosage first thing each morning. From there, I have them work up to a higher dose slowly until we find the right dosage for them.

Tribulus Terrestris

Healers around the world have used this little-known herb for centuries to treat sexual problems and to build muscle by boosting natural testosterone production. Oriental and Ayurvedic healers also used this herb to treat kidney, liver, and cardiovascular ailments.

Tribulus terrestris has been used in Turkish folk medicine to treat blood pressure. Healers in Europe have used it for centuries to treat sexual dysfunction, nervous disorders and headaches.[12] Bulgarian men used this same herb to improve sexual performance and heighten desire. Tests at the Bulgarian Medical Academy confirmed Tribulus terrestris to be an incredibly powerful aphrodisiac. When given to impotent and sexually disinterested animals, Tribulus terrestris caused them to begin active mating behavior and sexual intercourse.

Numerous animal studies confirm the usefulness of Tribulus terrestris as an aphrodisiac. Researchers in Singapore did a study on rats. They divided the rats into four groups: one control group and three groups receiving different doses of Tribulus terrestris ranging between 2.5 and 10 mg per kilogram of body weight. The study lasted 8 weeks. The researchers evaluated the rats for weight and sexual behavior. All the rats receiving Tribulus terrestris showed increased body weight and exhibited increased sexual behavior determined from an increase in mounting frequency. Rats receiving the highest doses of Tribulus terrestris had an average weight gain of 18% and a 24% increase in sexual behavior. Researchers attribute the changes to the herb's ability to increase androgen activity.[13]

In other animal studies Tribulus terrestris improves cardiovascular health. It lowered blood glucose by up to 40%. It lowered blood triglyceride levels by 23%, and it showed potential to lower cholesterol levels.[14] You may ask why this is relevant to your virility. Erectile dysfunction is often related to a problem with circulation—Tribulus terrestris increases your testosterone, and it may also improve your cardiovascular health, which can be surprisingly important for achieving and maintaining a healthy erection.

Studies with human patients offer more definitive support for the use of Tribulus terrestris to improve libido and sexual function. By gently boosting testosterone levels, Tribulus terrestris increases red blood cell counts, helping the body to transport oxygen, particularly in older men. Tribulus terrestris has been used in India for hundreds of years to help treat impotence and fatigue. In one study, 50 patients complaining of lethargy and fatigue for periods of two to six months were observed to show an overall improvement of 45% in all symptoms after taking Tribulus terrestris.

Tribulus terrestris also increases the blood levels of testosterone in healthy men by up to 30% in just five days of treatment.

Study after study shows that regular oral doses of Tribulus terrestris increase the testosterone levels of men suffering from impotence and infertility. It's one of my favorite herbs for men. By gently supporting your testosterone levels, Tribulus terrestris can help you to restore your strength, energy, and sexual desire to youthful levels.

Recommendation: 650 mg of Tribulus daily.

Yohimbine

Yohimbine comes from the inner bark of the Yohimbe tree that grows throughout Africa. It's long been considered an aphrodisiac, able to stimulate sexual desire and boost performance. This herb has been used in the United States for years to treat sexual problems in both men and women. Before pharmaceutical drugs, yohimbine was the only medication approved by the FDA for the treatment of impotence. Although the medical community has been divided on the therapeutic value of yohimbine, there seems little doubt that it has a restorative affect on sexual desire and erectile dysfunction in men. Yohimbine seems to work by preventing noradrenaline from stimulating a-adrenergic receptor sites. In other words, it helps keep your male hormones circulating longer. It's not clear whether it exerts its primary prosexual effect in the brain or in the penile arteries.

Many studies show the effectiveness of yohimbine in restoring sexual vigor in men. A review appearing in the *British Journal of Clinical Practice* examined the usefulness of yohimbine to treat erectile dysfunction. The author of this mainstream medical review reluctantly concluded that yohimbine does provide a therapeutic benefit in erectile dysfunction cases, especially those that are caused in part by a psychological issue. The review also found that yohimbine is well tolerated by most men.[15]

Another review of studies focused on seven studies that used randomized, placebo-controlled methods. Reviewers concluded that yohimbine is more than three times as effective as placebo treatments and rarely produces negative reactions. The reviewers state that for cases of erectile dysfunction, yohimbine should be tried before turning to pharmaceuticals.[16]

The most recent well-controlled study of yohimbine was conducted in Germany. A total of 83 men diagnosed with either organic or psychogenic erectile dysfunction took yohimbine (10mg, 3 times a day) or placebo for 8 weeks. The conclusion was an overall response rate of 71% for yohimbine versus only a 45% for placebo.

Recommendation: 250 mg of yohimbine extract daily.

Horny Goat Weed

Epimedium, or horny goat weed, is an ornamental herb found in both Asia and the Mediterranean. The traditional uses of horny goat weed include treating problems with the kidneys, liver, and joints. The most common historical uses are as an aphrodisiac and as an energy boost. Most of the research on the effectiveness of horny goat weed has been conducted in China and published in Chinese. Not all of these studies are available in English at this time, but the general conclusion is that horny goat weed effectively enhances sexual function.[17]

It's unclear exactly how horny goat weed works. Some researchers believe that it helps to lower cortisol levels, which as we saw earlier can ultimately lead to healthier testosterone levels by improving DHEA levels. Other researchers think it may increase the levels of neurotransmitters in the brain and some of these, like serotonin and dopamine, enhance sexuality, energy, and mood.

In one study conducted by doctors and the General Hospital of PLA in Beijing, China found that patients undergoing dialysis benefited from supplementing with horny goat weed. The patients taking horny goat weed experienced increased sexual function and improved quality of life versus patients with a similar health status that did not receive horny goat weed.[18] Another study examined the effect of icariin—a flavonoid present in horny goat weed—on erectile dysfunction. Icarrin was found to successfully inhibit PDE-5—the same mechanism that Viagra uses to help men with erectile dysfunction.[19]

Horny goat weed is safe when taken at recommended levels. It's certainly safer than taking a pharmaceutical, and I often recommend it to my patients needing help with erectile function.

Recommendation: 50 mg daily.

LongJax

The Tongkat Ali is a small tree that grows in Southeast Asia – also known as LongJax. Natives to Southeast Asia know it as a versatile, medicinal plant. One of its principle uses is as an aphrodisiac.

Studies that support LongJax's use as a aphrodisiac are primarily animal studies, but they are numerous and very promising.

For instance, middle-aged male mice receiving a daily supplement of LongJax showed increased sexual motivation within 10 days.[20] Another study found that middle-aged male rats given LongJax exhibited increased sexual behavior and libido.[21] Rats receiving LongJax were more likely to approach receptive females than those in the control groups and they were willing to go through more to reach females. LongJax rats would cross an electrified grid to reach female rats, while rats in the control group would not.[22]

In human studies, LongJax boosts muscle mass in men doing regular strength training. After five weeks of strength training, men taking LongJax supplements had significantly increased their lean muscle mass and strength when compared with men doing the same workouts but not taking LongJax. The LongJax group also reduced their body fat and their muscles were bigger than the control group.[23]

LongJax is safe to take, but it can cause insomnia and restlessness if you take doses that are too high for you. Since everybody is different, this can mean a little experimentation to find the dose that works best.

Recommendation: Start with a small dosage of 75 mg daily.

Citrulline

For many men, one of the most troublesome effects of declining testosterone and waning virility is the development of impotence or erectile dysfunction. In most cases, erectile dysfunction is a physical problem rather than a psychological one—only 10 to 20% of cases of erectile dysfunction are purely psychological in nature.[24]

Most erectile dysfunction is caused either by medications or a medical condition. There is a lot that has to happen for a successful erection to take place. The brain must receive stimulus and then react properly to it. Nerve impulses have to travel down the spinal column to the area around the penis. The muscles and nerves around the penis must relax properly to allow blood flow into the penis to create an erection, and adequate blood flow must be available. As you can see, there are a number of things involved. And if any one of these steps doesn't go *just right*, it can result in disappointment.

(We'll talk more about erectile dysfunction later in the book.)

Nitric oxide is one of the compounds critical to the relaxation of the muscles and arteries in the penis.

Arginine is an amino acid metabolized by the body into nitric oxide. Higher levels of circulating arginine can help with erectile dysfunction by helping the muscles within the penis to relax. At the University of Tel Aviv, researchers discovered that high doses of arginine taken daily by men experiencing erectile dysfunction can improve erections within two weeks.[25]

However, some researchers feel that another amino acid, *citrulline* may be even more effective at treating erectile dysfunction. Citrulline metabolizes into arginine in the body, and is readily released from the small intestine into circulation. Once circulating it is also readily converted into arginine by the kidneys.[26] Researchers at the East Caroline University conducted a clinical trial on patients with sickle cell disease. Patients received oral doses of L-Citrulline twice daily over the course of 4 weeks. The patients experienced a significant increase in their blood levels of arginine. The average arginine level increased by 65%.[27]

So, when it's arginine you're after, why take citrulline instead of going straight to the source? Well, it's a matter of absorption. Citrulline as a supplement absorbs into the body better than arginine. Researchers from the Anderson Cancer Center in Houston confirmed this when they found that rats given a diet supplemented with citrulline had higher plasma levels of arginine than those given a diet supplemented directly with arginine.[28]

Recommendation: Take 1000 mg daily for up to three months. (Individual amino acids shouldn't be taken for more than three months at a time— if you plan to use citrulline for longer than three months, add a balanced, mixed amino acid supplement as well)

L-Dopa

Dopamine is a chemical produced in your brain. It's vital for properly controlling your body movement. It also plays a role in that "feel-good" response you get from things like sex and food, which may be why l-dopa—a dopamine precursor—can increase libido.

The original application of l-dopa, which converts into dopamine in the brain, was to help treat Parkinson's disease. Soon after, it was recognized as a useful therapy for treating sexual dysfunction, as well. But it wasn't available except in prescription form… until it was discovered to have a natural source, that is.

Natural l-dopa can be extracted from the beans of the mucuna pruriens plant, and is available in non-prescription form. The libido-enhancing effects of l-dopa are proven in scientific studies. Because l-dopa's initial application was as a treatment for Parkinson's, it's not surprising that its potential for improving sexual dysfunction was first noticed among men with Parkinson's disease. Researchers found that sexual function improved significantly in patients taking a dopamine enhancer, especially in the younger men.[29]

L-dopa can have a powerful effect on your libido, but it's possible to overdo it. One case study reported in a Dutch medical journal discussed a man with Parkinson's disease who experienced periods of hypersexuality while taking prescription l-dopa. Though not life threatening, the episodes did interfere with the man's home care.[30] Thankfully, the natural form of l-dopa will gently enhance your sense of sexual desire without overwhelming you.

Recommendation: Take 300mg of natural l-dopa extract, (10% l-dopa) each day.

Secret #2

Don't Let Them Turn You into a Woman

Sideline the Chemicals Sabotaging Your Manhood

In Florida, alligator penises are shrinking. In fact, according to one researcher they "have such small penises that they are sexually incompetent."[1] And those poor gators aren't the only male animals having trouble: Male panthers have decreased sperm counts, the fertility of male bald eagles is decreasing, and male fish are showing feminine characteristics. The problems are not unique to Florida, either— it's happening all over the country.

None of this may sound like a big deal, but it affects you more than you might think. You see, the reason all these animals are having such a hard time is that they're being exposed to certain environmental chemicals—toxins that are sapping their virility. But here's the kicker: You're exposed to the same chemicals—every day. And the really bad news is you may be at an even higher risk than male wildlife because these chemicals have infiltrated almost every aspect of your life, including your food and water.

I'll tell you new ways to avoid, reduce, or eliminate your exposure to these chemicals so you can prevent them from making you fat, changing your brain chemistry, increasing your risk of impotence, and even shrinking your genitals.

When a Good Hormone Goes Bad

At the center of the problem, are chemicals that mimic estrogen. By chance or by fate, the molecular structure of these chemicals look almost identical to the hormone estrogen. When they get in your bloodstream, your body can't tell the difference.

As the imposter estrogens move through your body, they connect with receptors in your organs and other tissues. Once they get in, the cells in your body start to carry out the messages delivered by the fake hormones.

This can result in everything from early puberty to cancer or as in the case of the alligators – small penises.

Before you get the wrong idea, let me just say that not all estrogen is bad. Estrogen is the main female hormone, but even men naturally have small amounts of it in our bodies. Too much is bad news though—even in women (excessive estrogen causes cancer and other health problems in women). Men just are not supposed to have high levels of estrogen, which is exactly what environmental exposure to pesticides is causing.

But pesticides aren't the only sources of estrogen you're exposed to. Industries dump tons of pharmaceutical and synthetic estrogens that eventually seep into our drinking water.

And it doesn't stop there. Manufacturers line some food cans with estrogen-like compounds that blend with the food you eat. Manmade compounds used to manufacture plastics and even dental sealants in your mouth can mimic estrogen.

Cattle and poultry farms often use feeds that are high in estrogen. They do this because, just like us, farm animals fatten up from high levels of estrogen. But estrogens are some of the most stable ring structures in biology. So when you eat the meat from these animals, you're also eating some of the estrogen they ate.

All of this spells trouble for men.

Here's the Plain Truth: We Are Being Slowly Chemically Castrated

They say that the loss of testosterone is "natural," and some of it is. But in the 25 years that I've been studying the process of aging in men, I've discovered that a great deal of what some medical people accept as natural is, in fact, entirely *unnatural*.

Prostate cancer, for example. If you listened only to the AMA, you'd think that every man in every nation on earth gets prostate cancer at one time or another. The truth is shockingly different.

Prostate cancer is nearly entirely absent in parts of Asia and some third world countries. Prostate disease, in fact, appears to be largely the result of modern technology – the toxins we take into our body from artificial foods, from polluted air and contaminated water.

The same is true of many other forms of cancer. Heart disease, too.

You read more about these problems and their cures a little later in this book. For now, let's focus on how your environment is giving you feminine features without your consent.

<u>Male aging… and the reduction of testosterone related to it… is caused to a great degree by modern, artificial factors</u>.

Let's review some of them.

Water: A recent USGS study analyzing water samples found "… Traces of at least 11 compounds linked to birth control and hormone supplements."

Some studies have linked environmental exposure to hormones to deformed sex organs in wildlife, sex reversal in some fish and declining fertility in humans, as well as cancers and other diseases."

Meat and Poultry: In the old days, chickens went to market when they were about one year old. This is the natural amount of maturation required before a chicken can be slaughtered, sold and eaten.

Today, farmers cheat the natural growth process. They put growth stimulating hormones into the chicken feed. They dose baby chicks with dozens of growth stimulating hormones – mainly estrogens. Instead of the normal year they are quickly fattened up and sent to market at only *3 months* old! (Have you noticed how the texture and consistency of that the chicken breast you buy in the grocery has changed over the years?)

Incredibly, the FDA has maintained that the addition of hormones including estrogen mimicking compounds to our food is safe. Yet how could anyone know that this practice is safe? In other uses we are well And, the FDA and USDA do little to regulate the practice. In fact, they continue to approve new and more powerful hormones for farmers to use.

In 1990, the FDA ruled in favor of doubling the dose of hormones allowed in cattle. As if that weren't enough, many ranchers illegally implant more hormones into muscle tissue instead of the approve location behind the ear.

One study found that this illegal practice increases the level of estrogen in cattle – up to three-hundred times higher than what even the FDA approves.

Pesticides: Widely used pesticides interfere with male hormone production and mimic female hormones. Estrogen-like compounds also leak out of plastics, into our food, and eventually into us.

Over-Heating: The scrotum is not a design flaw. It has vital role in a man's health. It allows the testes to maintain a temperature a few degrees cooler than the rest of the body. This lower temperature is critical for normal testicular function. Unnaturally bind them up with jockey's or briefs... and they over-heat. This has been shown to significantly decrease testosterone production especially in older men.

Modern Day Stress: Any discussion of the assault of the modern world on testosterone would be incomplete without a pointing out the role of stress.

When we encounter danger in our path, our inborn response system activates. Hormones change, our pulse races, our breathing quickens and our muscles tense. Even our thinking speeds up. We either fight or run away and our physiology quickly returns to rest.

Today, we're exposed to sensations that prehistoric man never confronted. Pick up any newspaper. You'll find airplane crashes, earthquakes, famines and murder – more suffering than a man would have been exposed to in a lifetime a century ago. The difference is that we can't take action to resolve these crises. The result is unresolved chronic stress. <u>This unnatural stress suppresses testosterone.</u>

Drugs: Modern prescription drugs can have many side effects. Among the worst for men is their affect on testosterone. Some interfere with the production of testosterone others interfere with its actions. Even very common over the counter drugs can rob you of testosterone. (More on this later.)

These chemical estrogens are a lot tougher than you may think.

Being resistant to environmental breakdown, they can survive for decades without losing their punch. They are also highly fat-soluble. Once they get into your body, they live in your body's fat reserves.

Aside from being sturdy, they're able to link themselves to other chemical estrogens forming powerful combinations – an ability called *synergism*.[2]

Keep your Chest Looking Like a Man's

Unwanted effects vary from causing your prostate to swell to disrupting your urinary and reproductive systems to increasing your risk of testicular and prostate cancers. High estrogen levels can also wreak havoc on your mood, memory, mental clarity, and energy.

On top of all that, excess estrogen causes an extra layer of fat under your skin. This subcutaneous fat hides muscle definition and makes your body appear "doughy." And if you don't do anything about it, excess estrogen can cause gradual enlargement of your pectorals until they can resemble a woman's breasts.

If you go to a conventional doctor and complain of this problem, he'll probably send you to a plastic surgeon. They peel back your skin, remove the excess fat, and tack your nipple back in place. Of course, without diagnosing and addressing the underlying cause, the breasts just grow back.

But there are steps you can take to prevent any and all of this from happening to you.

Your Step-by-Step Guide for Lowering Estrogen

For starters, I recommend that you ask your doctor to measure the "total estrogens" in your blood. On the same sample, ask him to measure your testosterone as well. Your blood test will provide critical information regarding the ratio between your estrogen and testosterone.

For most of my male patients, I want a ratio of at least four parts testosterone per one part estrogen. For maximal "manpower," I want eight times more testosterone than estrogen. Sometimes in athletes we shoot for a 10 to 1 ratio. It's also important for you to keep your total estrogen level below 100.

Once you've figured out your current "baseline," take the following steps to reverse the hormonal sabotage those environmental chemicals are inflicting on your sexual health.

• Eliminate pesticides from your water: I recommend drinking only purified water.

• Wash your vegetables and fruits before you eat them.

• Cut off any visible fat from meat before cooking since chemicals and hormones from the feed collect in the fat.

• Avoid processed meats, because they have fat ground in.

• Avoid processed carbohydrates like bread, cereals, and pasta. They make your body release excess insulin, which builds fat and stimulates feminizing estrogen.

• Eat vegetables high in fiber to keep yourself regular. When stool remains in your bowel for a longer time, more estrogen is absorbed.[3]

- Eat more cruciferous vegetables like broccoli, cauliflower, Brussels's sprouts, and cabbage. They help you excrete excess estrogen.

- Eat hormone-free food and free range animals whenever possible.

- Incorporate more estrogen-inhibiting foods into your diet. Some of the best and tastiest sources are squash, onions, green beans, cabbage, berries, citrus, pineapples, pears, grapes, figs, melons, sesame seeds, and pumpkin seeds.[4]

- Cut back on alcohol and work with your doctor to reduce your medication dosages as much as possible. These things interfere with liver function and you need your liver operating up to par so it can remove those excess estrogens from your system ASAP.

To rid your body of excess estrogen, here are two additional tools: The first is a plant compound called indole-3-carbinol (I3C). The other estrogen-regulating tool is diindolylmethane or DIM. *(See Secret #1 for more details.)*

Both of these compounds are readily available in supplement form at nutrition stores.

Make the Most of Your Manhood

The bottom line is you don't have to stand by and watch while your manhood (in every sense of the word) shrivels up. You don't have to follow in the footsteps of the alligators in Florida. Take the steps outlined above to reverse environmental estrogen's signal to turn you into a woman. It's an important step to keep you strong and virile in our modern world.

Secret #3

Eat Food Fit for a Man

The Biggest Con of Our Time

For 30 years, the American Heart Association, the modern food industry and the media have been telling you the secret to good health is a low-fat diet.

This is a dangerous mistake.

For years, a handful of us in medicine have been telling you the opposite—that dietary fat is not the problem. And when you eat low-fat, you inevitably eat more carbohydrate and inadvertently sacrifice the most important nutrient, protein. This is the prescription for losing vital muscle and turning your body into flab.

All along, we've had a growing body of medical studies backing up our claims. But the governmental organizations have stubbornly clung to their low-fat hypothesis and the mainstream media have failed to recognize the mounting evidence against it.

A few years ago, *The New York Times Sunday Magazine* ran a cover story entitled "What If It's All Been a Big Fat Lie?" The article said the American medical establishment's worst nightmare had come true—not only had they been wrong about what constitutes a healthy diet, but their recommendations had made the problem worse… and their critics had been right all along.

In this secret, you'll see how to take that long-overdue "revelation" a step farther. You'll learn why eating a low-fat, high-carb diet not only makes you fatter, but also puts you at risk for a slew of medical problems—from the onset of diabetes to heart disease and stroke.

You'll also learn:

• How starches make you fat.

• How protein makes you strong and healthy.

• Why eating some fat is essential for good health.

• Why cholesterol is not the threat that you've been told.

In short, you'll be able to fuel your body with the natural foods you were meant to eat. Losing weight will come easier and faster. You will be able to build a masculine V-taper. And you will wake-up feeling charged with energy that will last the whole day.

Eat Food You Can Sink Your Teeth Into

The New York Times Magazine article was largely correct. Hundreds of medical studies have shown that the low-fat, high-starch diet advocated by so many has made American men fatter, sicker and less... well, manly.

If you want to live a long healthy life, you have to forget about tofu burgers and whole grain breads. The good news is you can start eating the foods you like. You can eat the things your father probably told you would "put hair on your chest" decades ago – like steak and eggs!

I've already helped hundreds of men use this approach. I've seen them make the transformation from fat and sickly to lean and healthy. My clinic is full of patients who used to take multiple medications and now take none. Along with becoming lean, these men see their cholesterol and triglycerides drop, their high blood pressures resolve, their pain of arthritis gone and their diabetes reversed.

Our Wellness Research Foundation has collected compelling scientific evidence that not only the modern epidemic of obesity but many "modern" diseases are either caused or worsened by following the diet that you've been told was healthy.

There is still much to be learned about nutrition. But one thing is becoming increasingly clear. The best diet for men is the diet that men instinctively want to eat. It's the diet we were eating – without the help of modern medicine – for eons.

Let's look at the facts.

What Did Adam Really Eat?

The earliest evidence of the diet of early man comes from fossils. The record is unambiguous. Early man preferred animal flesh. His whole culture was built around acquiring and consuming meat.

And we can go even further back in time. Man's closest living relative, the chimpanzee regularly hunts down and consumes animal flesh. The meat is very highly prized, with the highest-ranking members consuming their fill first. They show a preference for the fat and the organs of their prey.

When all those vegetarian books were so popular back in the 60's and 70's, primatologists believed most other primates were vegetarians. This was cited as a reason why we should all swear off beef and eat bean sprouts instead. I still see this claim being made but we now know it to be false. Most other primates regularly eat insects, forage for small animals and routinely hunt down and eat any game they can kill.

There Are No Native Vegetarians

Perhaps even more convincing, is the data from indigenous cultures. Many of these cultures survived unaffected by the modern world into the 20th century. Anthropologists studied and recorded their dietary habits.

Of particular note is the work of Dr. Weston Price. He traveled throughout the world meticulously documenting their lifestyles. He studied 14 remaining hunter-gatherer cultures.

He discovered two very remarkable features in every culture. One, they were universally lean and lacked the modern constellation of diseases. Two, they all prized and ate meat. There was not a single vegetarian culture.

An extensive study of the health of native people was conducted by Dr. Loren Cordain. Dr. Cordain is an expert on primitive dietary habits and a professor of exercise physiology at Colorado State University. He examined the diets of 229 of the worlds remaining native societies. Here's a summary of his findings.

• He also found no vegetarian cultures.

• Game as their principal source of protein and fat.

• Hunted game or fish was highly valued.

• Organ meat was most coveted, often reserved for the privileged.

Dr. Cordain also found hunter-gatherers relied on animal products as their main food source. Animal foods make up 50-65% of the societies' diets. Cordain concluded:

"... this high reliance on animal-based foods coupled with the relatively low carbohydrate content of wild plant foods produces universally characteristic macronutrient consumption ratios in which protein intakes are greater at the expense of carbohydrate." [1]

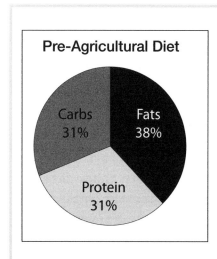

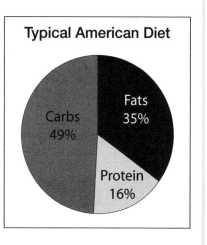

The fact that native pre-agricultural societies universally ate more protein than the average modern diet surprises my patients. They have read that we eat too much protein.

The evidence when taken together makes one conclusion undeniable. A vegetarian diet has never been the natural diet of man. The truth is the exact opposite. For millions of years man has eaten meat. What's more, meat was universally prized in every primitive culture.

Natives Who Ate Higher Protein Were Healthier

Politically correct or not, the more meat an endogenous society ate, the healthier it appeared. For instance, the Masai of east Africa who live on raw milk, cattle meat and blood and organ meat appeared to completely lack dental cavities, obesity or heart disease.

Among the healthiest of all native groups studied are the Dinkas. They live along the banks of the Nile River and live mostly on fish and shellfish. One western physician who lived among them reported to have never seen a single case of obesity, heart disease or cancer in 15 years.

The Beginning of the Problem

10,000 years ago, people began to domesticate plants and animals. There was a gradual switch from hunting and gathering to farming. Farming could support a larger population. Quality was sacrificed for the sake of quantity. This was the start of the Agricultural Revolution.

Archaeologists can identify the Agricultural Revolution in the fossil record. Human remains tell the tale of the agriculture. But not in the way you might think. Skeletal relics can show the age, gender, height, weight, illnesses, and the state of health of an individual. Archaeologists have found that farming communities were more malnourished and disease ridden than their hunter-gatherer predecessors.

Hunter-gatherer skeletons in Greece show that the average height was about 5'9". That was until the advent of agriculture, then the Greeks suddenly shrank to a mere 5'. Even today, the Greek population has not fully regained the height of their primitive predecessors.

The record of native people in the Illinois and Ohio River valleys also demonstrate the health consequences of agriculture.

"Archaeologists have excavated some 800 skeletons that paint a picture of the health changes that occurred when a hunter-gatherer culture gave way to the intensive maize farming around A. D. 1150 … these early farmers paid a price for their new-found livelihood. Compared to the hunter-gatherers who proceeded them, the farmers had a nearly 50% increase … in malnutrition, a fourfold increase in iron-deficiency anemia …[and] a threefold rise in infectious disease." [2]

Farmers always grow high-carbohydrate crops. There are no other crops. Even the soybean often touted for is high protein is still over 80% carbohydrate. Other staple crops like potatoes, corn, wheat, and rice are all over 90% carbohydrate.

Farming communities no longer receive the range of nutrients that hunters-gatherers had. And, farmers do not consume high amounts of protein. Malnourished farmers were more susceptible to disease.

The record is consistent. When hunter-gatherers switched to farming, their protein intake went down and their carbohydrate intake went up. The incidence of malnutrition and diseases rose in every case I can find.

Of course, the sudden rise in the modern constellation of diseases did not go unnoticed. In the middle of the last century, it began to be identified as the modern plague.

The problem is the archaeological record was not as complete as it is today. Nutrition was a fledgling science. The medical establishment identified only single nutrient deficiencies as causes of disease. It was very slow to accept nutrition as a fundamental basis of good health. The reasons conspired to produce what I consider to be the biggest mistake in the history of nutrition.

Science Takes Wrong Turn

You can blame a reductionist view of health, you can blame the commercial interest of food producers or slick Madison Avenue marketing but for one reason or another, the cause of the problem was misread.

Without real evidence, fat was identified as the culprit. It was not known that native diets ate more fat than modern diets. Endocrinology or the study of hormones was not considered.

If we can divorce ourselves from the prejudice about fat, the endocrinology is really quite simple. Your body controls fat building. Hormones are used to set the controls. The hormone insulin controls fat.

How much insulin do you secrete in response to a fat laden meal? Zero. Insulin is secreted in response to carbohydrate. Eat more carbohydrate and you will secrete more insulin and build more fat all other things being equal. Fat in the diet, in contrast, is neutral.

Scientists have even recently identified the cellular machinery that turns carbohydrates into fat. Researchers at the University of Texas Southwestern Medical Center found a protein in cells called ChREBP. It converts excess dietary carbohydrates into fat stores.

Over Consumption of Carbohydrate Gets Worse

In 1977, George McGovern led a Senate Committee that released its "Dietary Goals for the United States". The publication advised that Americans drastically cut their dietary fat intake. And, according to the "Dietary Goals", fat was the cause of illnesses sweeping the nation.

The National Institutes of Health jumped on the "ban fat" wagon. In 1984, NIH announced that Americans must cut their fat intake. In response, the food industry quickly produced a slew of "low-fat" products. But without the tasty fat, the food produced was bland. High amounts of sugar became a common additive.

Americans replaced fat with refined carbohydrates and sugar. The amount of calories from fat in the American diet decreased. And, the amount of calories from refined carbohydrates increased... dramatically.

Cereals were cheap to produce and could be sold at a huge profit. When Kellogg and other early proponents of cereals started their health farms, they preached that modern society was oversexed. Eating cereal they claimed would solve the problem.

As bizarre as this and the other inflated and unsubstantiated claims were, there might be a twisted kernel of truth. Cholesterol is the building block for testosterone. If you deprive yourself of animal fat, your testosterone will go down.

As you saw in Secret #1, testosterone deficiency has the worst kinds of consequences for men – impotence, depression, obesity and fatigue to name a few. I've seen evidence for this, first hand. Some of the most severe testosterone deficiencies I've encountered were in men eating very low-fat diet. Often, they had gotten this advice from their physicians.

Some Fat Is Essential

The main problem I have with low fat is that it also means high carb. Excessive intake of carbohydrate is the central dietary problem in my patient population. But there is another problem emerging from the low-fat advice. The lower fat intake itself can be detrimental to your health.

One study published in the *Journal of Clinical Nutrition* found that low-fat diets affect calcium absorption. The study found low-fat diets were associated with 20% lower calcium absorption than higher fat diets.[3]

The State University of New York at Buffalo also found that low-fat diets cause health problems. The researchers found that people who eat low-fat diets develop weaker immune systems.[4]

Another study examined people eating very low fat diets, (14% fat). People eating very low fat diets showed no improvement in body composition, blood sugar levels, insulin levels, or blood pressure levels. The study's authors called very low fat diets "counterproductive" to health. [5]

A certain amount of fat is critical to absorb vitamins. The fat-soluble nutrients like vitamins A, D, E, and K and coenzyme CoQ10 cannot be absorbed without fat.

The Solution: Using Modern Science to Emulate the Past

The good news is that fixing this mess is not as hard as you might think. What was caused by 10 millennia of farming and worsened by weak science and bad advice can be fixed by you alone.

And don't be worried that eating meat is going to drive up your cholesterol.

A number of studies have also been done concerning lean meat and cholesterol. One of the most recent studies has proven that the incorporation of lean meat into the diet helps reduce cholesterol levels. By the way, it didn't matter whether it was white meat and red meat. Both lowered bad LDL cholesterol and raised good HDL cholesterol. [6]

Numerous studies have proven that low-carbohydrate diets improve diabetes. One important study analyzed diabetic patients for 8 weeks. Some of the patients ate a diet with 55% of calories from carbohydrates (very similar to the average American's diet). The other group ate a diet where 25% of the calories came from carbohydrates. The group eating the 25% diet experienced a drop in blood sugar levels. People eating the 55% diet experienced a rise in blood sugar levels. Those eating more carbohydrates worsened their diabetic condition. [7]

The *Journal of Nutrition* published a German study that proved the importance of protein. The researchers found that high protein diets boost antioxidant levels. The higher the protein consumed, the higher the antioxidant levels became. Low protein consumption actually seemed to induce the oxidative affects of free radicals.[8]

An alarming report out of Stockholm University has raised even more debate about carbohydrates. The report, released through Sweden's National Food Administration, found cancer-causing agents in breads, rice, potatoes, and cereals. Starch transforms into a compound called acrylamide when heated. Acrylamide is a known carcinogen and recognized by the US Environmental Protection Agency. [9]

Secret #4

Make More Manly Muscle

Use It or Lose It!

Let's step back and consider a broader perspective on the issue of exercise.

In an idyllic existence, you really shouldn't have to exercise. You should be perfectly adapted so that your level of activity is exactly what you need to keep you at your best function. The problem here is that our current activity in our modern world has completely changed from the native activity and physical challenges that produced our physical adaptations.

Since we are no longer using our bodies for the hunting prey, defending against predators and fighting for dominance that it was designed for, another feature of our adaptability comes into prominence. If we don't use a physical capacity, our bodies are designed to no longer expend the metabolic machinery necessary to build and maintain that feature and we gradually lose it.

Exercise then becomes necessary to prevent or reverse losses caused by disuse.

So if you exclude the use of exercise for the purpose of enhancing sports performance or boosting a capacity beyond its native level... and focus on exercising for good health ... three guiding principles follow. They may seem obvious when they are spelled out but nonetheless, I have yet to see a single exercise program that consciously addresses them.

First off, it should prevent or reverse a loss of a physical attribute or capacity that you consider desirable.

Secondly, it should reproduce or mimic an activity that you would have performed routinely in your native habitat but is not required in your current environment.

Thirdly, the more you have altered your environment the more you need an exercise program. (Think of the known consequences of a hospitalized patient or an astronaut in space not exercising.) And conversely, if you can reincorporate an activity in your environmental routine you may eliminate the need for that type of exercise challenge.

This last principle is a little known key to your long-term health. Think of your exercise program as the leading edge of your use of your intelligence and strength of will to change your body. Then, you should continually strive to roll that challenge into your recreation, sport, work or other routine activities.

So a well-rounded fitness strategy identifies physical losses and mimics our now missing but native challenges from our hunter past to rebuild the lost capacity. Unfortunately, most modern exercise routines you've heard about do not do this.

In fact, most of what you have learned about fitness and exercise is inaccurate, incomplete or downright dangerous.

For instance, traditional "cardio" by running long distances or spending hours on the treadmill actually decreases your heart capacity. In addition, endurance training actually encourages your body to produce more fat while burning away your muscle.

What's more, traditional weight training forces us to use unnatural body movements that can produce injury and pain. Weight training can produce increases in muscle mass but is not well designed to build strength.

Size Is Important – But It's Not the Only Thing

Let's get one thing straight, I often see confused. **Muscle size and strength are not the same things**. Yea, of course the two are related but modern day body builders create so much muscular hypertrophy that they can hardly get out of their own way.

In contrast, some guys need to increase the size of their muscles. In that case, resistance training may be the best course. It is a scientific way to apply overload to isolate muscles. Since you can easily manipulate the resistance by incrementally increasing the weight, you can perpetuate the stimulus for muscle growth.

Muscle wasting has its consequences in aging. If you do lift weights you should measure and focusing on your muscle size as the goal. Don't confuse it with functional strength in real world situations.

But in years of practical application, one glaring limitation of weight training remains. It's not really "training" anything. It's more "untraining" your muscles. It teaches them to do nothing but tense. And there are other problems….

The Rugged Truth about Weight Training

Weight training will not produce overall body fitness or the functional strength, energy and stamina you need. Weights work well to build muscle mass and sometimes guys either need or want that. But do not confuse size with real world strength.

You can get a set of bulging biceps and chest to tense into stoic poses if that's what you want. But typical weight training often leads to chronic injuries in weight trainers. Here some of the problems:

1. Weight training unnaturally isolates the development of individual muscles weakening stabilizing muscles critical for proper posture and maximum strength.

2. Weight training causes repetitive stress injuries of the tendons and ligaments.

3. It encourages hairline and stress related bone fractures.

4. It drastically increases chronic rotator cuff injuries of the shoulder.

5. It promotes anterior shoulder instability eventually positioning the shoulder forward. This is important: If you practice typical weight training pressing movements, you will very likely develop chronic shoulder pain.

6. Over time, virtually all heavy lifters experience some level of chronic pain in the knees, back, elbows, wrists or shoulders.

It's not that taxing your muscles is bad. On the contrary challenging your muscles under tension is the only way to increase muscle mass. It's just that most weight training uses stresses not encountered in our natural environment. It will eventually lead to more pain than gain.

Weight training tends to isolate a single muscle group. It places you on a bench or in a rack or instructs you not to allow other parts of your body to move. This places too much stress on isolated muscles while leaving critical stabilizing muscles completely untrained.

If you want real strength – strength you can use everyday – there is a better way.

Cave Man Calisthenics

The best way to build real functional strength is to practice exercises that put your body through natural patterns of movement. Traditionally, we call these exercises calisthenics. The word comes from ancient Greece. The ancient Greeks knew that by running sprinting races, wrestling, and performing a series of calisthenics they were able to achieve a level of physical strength and beauty we still revere today....and they are still the best way to build functional strength.

Calisthenics are also much more effective in strengthening ligaments and tendons. And, by doing regular calisthenics, you will be lowering your risk of injury and building muscle that has been trained for function.

That's why in almost every military tradition you'll find extensive use of calisthenics. In fact, many of the most elite Special Forces troops in the field today rely heavily on these simple exercises to remain in top-notch physical condition no matter where they are.

With improved functional strength, you will

find greater ease in performing routine physical tasks. What's more, you can do calisthenics at home, in the office or while you are on the road.

What's more, repeatedly exercising in short duration sessions retrains your body to store energy for fast access. In addition, compact exercise routines force your body to burn fat during the muscle recovery process.

You can do them in short bursts of 10-minutes or less. They do not require expensive equipment. You can do them anywhere or anytime. And, you can exercise muscle groups in the patterns of movement that fit their designed purpose. Since they are intended to mimic natural challenges, the maneuvers are simple, instinctive and easy to learn.

Exercises that put your body through natural patterns of movement also train your entire circuit from thought to action. This "neuromuscular education" is essential if you want that new muscle to be capable of doing anything.

Before beginning any exercise program, check with your doctor to make sure that it's safe for you. Especially if you have had health problems or your family has a history of heart trouble. Secondly, when beginning an exercise program, it's important to start out light and increase your effort over time.

To Strengthen Your Base - Go to Where the Muscle Is

Let's start from the bottom up. In building strength you want to work the big muscles first. Your biggest muscles are the quadriceps on the front of your thigh followed by the hamstrings group on the back of your thigh. These big muscles lose their strength if you don't challenge them.

The lower body is also more important than the upper body for maintaining your strength later in life. Having muscular shoulders, chest and arms looks great at the beach but having a muscular imbalance between your chest and arms and your lower body causes more harm than good to functional strength. And, it puts excess pressure on your joints and weakens your posture over time.

Alternating Lunges: Stand straight with your hands on your hips and feet together. Take a long step forward with your left leg and bring your right knee down to the ground. Now bring your right leg forward and return to a standing position. Repeat. (Try these in a hallway, since you'll be moving forward a few feet each time.)

Squats: With your feet at shoulder width and pointing slightly away from each other, move your buttocks down and backward as if you were about to sit on a low stool. The key is to keep your knees from extending beyond your toes. Keep moving downward until your thighs are parallel to the floor. Keep your back straight. It's best not to squat with your heels raised. This stresses the ligaments in your knees.

Squat Leaps: Now for a more challenging strength builder. Stand straight with your hands on your hips and feet apart at shoulder width. Squat down until your legs are almost at right angles, then jump straight up as high as you can. Pretend you're a rocket launching. This exercise will put a spring in your step.

Strengthen Your Center of Power

Now let's concentrate on your abdomen. You can't have functional strength without a strong core. Mid-section strength improves breath, posture and mechanics of motion. Strong abdominal muscles also help prevent injury to your lower back.

Remember though, these exercises won't eliminate your spare tire. The exercises for the large muscles of the legs along with cutting down on carbs will do more for thinning down your waist.

Crunches: Here's a group of exercises that you can vary to continue to challenge your mid-section strength. Start by lying on your back. Place your palms on the floor and move your hands underneath your buttocks. Slowly raise your head and feet slightly off the ground, hold for 1 second and slowly lower them. Repeat.

I like the *Official United States Navy SEAL Workout,* which uses several variations of crunches. Not all of them require you to touch your thighs with your elbows. You may find this hard to accomplish and it's not essential. You can do them raising only your head or your entire torso as in a sit-up. You can do them raising your feet slightly off the ground or straight up in the air. You can do them with one leg crossed over the other at the knee.[3]

Leg Levers: Starting from six inches above the ground, lift them about another foot higher and bring them back down to the starting position. Repeat.

Back Flutter Kicks: Alternate raising each leg from the starting position to about two or three feet off the ground.

Scissors: Again from the starting position, raise your legs a few inches off the ground. Now spread your legs apart and bring them back together. Repeat. Your legs will look like a pair of scissors opening and closing.

Build Balanced Strength in Your Chest and Arms

Body-building enthusiasts often limit their functionality and range of motion by "over sizing" a few select muscles of their upper bodies. When you do work your upper body, you should focus on your back more than your chest and arms. Again, use the principle of "work big muscles first". If you use your own body weight as resistance, you will not only build strength for those exercises, but you will also power your ability to do everyday activities like lifting a heavy package or moving a couch. Your muscle will be useful to you instead of just eye candy for the ladies.

Pushups: I am very fond of the basic push-up. My father taught them to my before kindergarten. If I had only one upper body exercise this would be it. They work your entire upper body. They strengthen the pectorals of the chest, the deltoids of the shoulders, the triceps of the arms and the muscles of the upper, mid and lower back.

By the way, bench presses are poor substitutes for pushups. The mechanics are different. In a bench press, your shoulder blade presses flat against the bench and is unable to move putting all of the stress on the shoulder joint. This is one of the major reasons most weight lifters eventually develop anterior shoulder problems.

Your hands should set a little wider than shoulder width, your feet should be together, and your back should be straight. Lower yourself until you're almost touching the ground. If you're having trouble with these at first, try doing them with your knees on the ground and your feet in the air. If you can handle pushups well, here's an additional challenge: See if you can clap your hands between pushups.

Arm Haulers: After you're done with your pushups, you might get tired and will want to lie on your stomach for a while. While you're down there, try this exercise. Stretch your arms in front of you, and raise your arms and legs off the floor. Then sweep your arms all the way back to your thighs -- like you're doing the breaststroke -- and bring them back to the starting position. This is great for the back and shoulders.

Pull-ups: These you do with your palms facing out. With basic pull-ups, you will strengthen the muscles of the middle back. You can vary the width of your grip on the bar -- a wide grip really widens your back for more a V-taper. You can change your grip to palm facing you for a chin-up. They're a little easier to do than pull-ups. They also strengthen your back but recruit your biceps as well.

Dips: You can do these between two chairs or two desks or a set of parallel bars. While putting one hand on each object, lift your feet off the ground; then slowly lower yourself until your elbows are about at a 90-degree angle then come back up more slowly. This exercise is great for the chest, middle back and triceps.

Remember to start out slowly. If you do the exercises consistently and stay with the program, you could see results in just a few weeks.

Now, Why You Can't Ignore Size

Right now, you are losing a vital asset for virility and youth: your muscle.

Unless you stop it, you will lose muscular strength and mass as you age. And, contrary to popular belief, science is showing that muscle actually becomes even more important as you grow older. Unfortunately, most doctors completely ignore this problem. They wait until it has produced serious health consequences and then prescribe drugs for the symptoms.

Loss of youthful muscle is responsible for many of the other unhealthy changes we see with aging. It not only causes weakness and fatigue but also fat gain, apathy, sexual dysfunction, chronic illness, bone fractures, depression, sagging skin and multiple hormonal declines have all been linked to loss of muscle.

Fortunately, you don't have to accept muscle deterioration with all its consequences. You can restore 100 % of your youthful muscle mass. In doing so, you restore virility, power, drive, and abilities of your youth.

In this chapter, I'll show you new evidence that reveals why building muscle is so important. I'll also give you my advice on the best food, supplements and exercise for achieving and maintaining peak muscle mass and strength.

Muscle is Youth: The Untold Story

When I teach anatomy and physiology to college students, I stump them with the question "What are the functions of muscle?" Most students can only give me one; muscle moves your body. But muscle does so much more than that. Your body's muscles form a complex interconnected organ. It stores energy, regulates metabolism and generates vital feedback control to hormone production.

Your muscle is responsible for a wide array of body functions. Here are just some of the most important.

Benefits of Healthy Muscle

Improves sexual health by stimulating sexual hormone production	**Preserves youth** by stimulating human growth hormone
Reduces risk of bone fractures by supporting bones	**Keeps you trim** by boosting your metabolic rate
Decreases risk of disease by strengthening your immune system	**Gives you more energy** by storing more glycogen

In addition to being an anti-aging physician, I am also a personal trainer. This combination has given me a special appreciation of the value of muscle in reversing many of the consequences of aging. I see men in their 60s, 70, and 80s who think that muscle is no longer important. But they couldn't be more wrong.

When I see these patients for the first time, I perform body composition tests on them. This way I can tell how much of their body is made of fat and muscle. Older men often measure dangerously low percentages of muscle.

The Measure of Generations

You begin losing muscle around the age of 30. Every decade after that you lose about 3 pounds of muscle – unless you do something about it. Many people blame their weakness, fat gain, and sluggishness on "just getting older". But it's largely due to the decrease in muscle and its effects on the body. And, that is reversible.

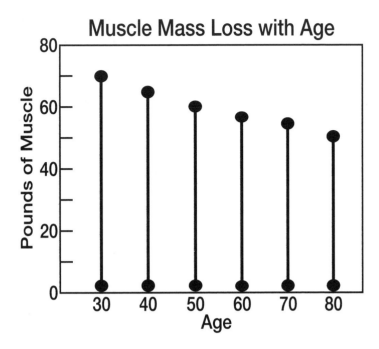

This muscle loss with age has a medical term: sarcopenia. Sarcopenia literally means "loss of flesh." There is growing evidence linking sarcopenia with:

- Functional disability

- Glucose intolerance

- Decreased physical activity

- Oxidative stress

- Derangement of normal hormone production[1]

Most importantly, sarcopenia causes weakness. This leads to the loss of the capacity to perform activities of daily living. It is a major cause of the nursing home institutionalization of so many elder Americans. And it is the biggest cause of falls in elders.

I believe sarcopenia is the root cause of more fractures in men than osteoporosis.

Regaining Your Youth

Muscle loss is not inevitable. Your age doesn't have to dictate your health. We have proven that even very elder nursing home residents can restore their youthful muscle mass. You can build back 100% of your muscle with the right techniques.

For 20 years I have observed and measure muscle's youth preserving effects. Now I have more supporting evidence. An ongoing Finnish study called the Evergreen Project is currently studying the effects of muscle on the aging process. Men and women between the ages of 65 and 94 are participating in the study.

The study is proving wide-ranging benefits that go hand in hand with muscle building. Results show that the participants with the most muscle are experiencing better mental function, fewer chronic illnesses, and longer life spans.[2]

When I see that a new patient is suffering from muscle loss, I immediately put them on a muscle-building plan. The plan is simple. I give them a program to optimize their nutrition and exercise to put them on a road to build back the muscle of their youth. Here are the most important features for you to benefit from the muscle of your youth.

Important Exercise for Building Muscle

Exercise is, of course, the key to preserving muscle. But probably not in the way you are thinking. When I measure muscle mass in my clinic and prescribe building X pounds of muscle back, nearly everyone thinks of gym exercises for the arms, chest and shoulders. Yes, that can build some muscle, but it can't address the consequences of age-associated sarcopenia. Here's why:

Your upper extremities only contain about 15% of your body's muscle mass. You can increase their size by 200% and yet I will barely be able to measure a difference in your body's total muscle mass. To affect this number, you must go where the big muscles are.

The biggest muscles in the body are the quadriceps on the front of your thighs. The second largest are the gluteus muscles in your buttocks, and third are the hamstrings on the back of your thighs. Therefore, your most important anti-aging, muscle-restoring exercises must flex and extend the hip joint.

Another important principle for building muscle is to do the compound (moving more than one joint) and heaviest exercises at the beginning of your workout. Work your large muscle groups first; i.e., your legs and back. You can do any exercise that provides sufficient resistance over a wide enough range of motion for the large muscles of the legs and back.

For most men the fastest muscle-building workout is a split routine. This means that you don't perform the same exercises every time you work out. You split the exercises into 2 groups done on different days.

You also need a cardiopulmonary activity. Avoid long-term cardiovascular exercises. This can actually strip you of muscle. Cardio endurance activities like jogging will burn off your well-earned muscle.

What you need instead is activity to support peak cardiopulmonary function. My PACE® program will give your heart and lungs the workout they need without stripping you of muscle. For cardiopulmonary capacity, remember to include your P.A.C.E. program in your regimen. You can find descriptions of P.A.C.E. programs at my website at: www.AlSearsMD.com

Testosterone: Muscle building in men would not be complete without addressing testosterone. Testosterone tells your body to become manly and produce lean muscle mass. If your levels of testosterone are low, your body will find it harder to build muscle.

I always check a man's testosterone levels if he is trying to gain muscle. Often a combination of herbal testosterone boosters dramatically improves muscle gains. If your levels are low, go back to secret 1, and follow the advice for boosting testosterone.

Designing a Workout Plan

Try to decide on some favorites and then create your program. The different patterns of exercises you can do are countless. I like to do 3 sets of 10 for each exercise I choose for the day. Split up your exercise by major muscle groups.

My Favorite Workout Plan:

Day 1	Abs and Legs
Day 2	Back, Chest, Shoulders and Arms
Day 3	P.A.C.E.
Day 4	Abs and Legs
Day 5	Back, Chest, Shoulders and Arms
Day 6	P.A.C.E.
Day 7	Rest

How to Use Muscle and Strength Building Nutrients

You can't build muscle if you don't give it the nourishment it needs. A high protein diet and the right supplements will increase the effectiveness of muscle-building exercises. Here are some of the best nutrients. They are proven by the trial and error of athletes and by controlled scientific studies. They'll give your body the boost it needs to become a muscle-building machine.

Protein: The change here is simple. Eat more protein. Protein constitutes muscle. Your body needs excess protein to support new muscle growth. The best sources of muscle-building protein are lean red meat, fish, eggs, milk, cheese, beans and nuts. Make sure that protein is the main course of every meal. Throw out the carbohydrate snacks and snack on boiled eggs, nuts, sliced turkey breasts and nuts instead.

Creatine: Supplements can also help your body to build muscle. One of the safest and best-researched supplements to increase muscle mass and strength is creatine. Creatine increases sports performance, endurance, strength and speed and will increase the muscle you build during resistance training.

One recent study analyzed 28 healthy participants over the age of 65. Half of the participants took creatine, while the other half took a placebo. All of the subjects followed the same weight-training program for 4 weeks. The participants taking creatine had a larger increase in muscle mass than those taking the placebo.[3] I recommend taking 5 mg of creatine daily until you build the muscle you need.

L-Arginine: Another supplement for muscle building is the essential amino acid, L-arginine. One double-blinded study measured the change in muscle strength and lean muscle mass in men taking L-arginine.

Twenty-two men on a strength-training program took either the L-arginine supplement or a placebo. The men taking the arginine supplement showed a significant increase in muscle strength and lean muscle mass after only 5 weeks.[4] I have used arginine-containing supplements for 20 years. Like creatine, it is natural and safe. From 500 mg to 1g of L-arginine will support muscle growth.

Carnosine: Carnosine is a multi-functional substance made from two amino acids. Carnosine is naturally present in your nerve and muscle cells. Carnosine protects the integrity of the muscle you have, and the muscle you are building.

I recommend taking 500 mg of carnosine, twice a day. You need carnosine to ensure that the muscle you are trying to build will be healthy and last.

Glutamine: The amino acid glutamine is an important muscle-building supplement for a couple of reasons. For starters, glutamine helps to stabilize your energy levels. But more importantly, glutamine actually boosts the natural growth hormone in your body. Growth hormone tells your body to shed fat and build muscle. In addition, I use glutamine in athletes to prevent muscle breakdown.

Doctors have now begun to use glutamine to reduce muscle loss in cancer patients. Cancer patients often have severe muscle breakdown. A recent study showed that a glutamine cocktail actually helped cancer patients to reverse their muscle loss.[5]

For maximal muscle growth, take glutamine as a powder at 5 grams per day. You can dissolve it in water or put it in a protein shake.

Now for your last little-know secret to keeping manly function and form – a better way to maintain your most important ranges of motion.

Stay Limber at Any Age

As you age certain muscles shorten you lose range of motion. Routine daily activities become intimidating challenges. I've treated patients who no longer had the free movement they needed to dress themselves. This doesn't have to be your fate.

An intelligent stretching regimen can prevent or reverse this condition. The real solution is simple, pleasant and takes only a couple of minutes. Yet the advice you see on stretching is time-consuming and boring. It's sometimes contradictory and in many cases more harmful than helpful. I often see programs to "stretch out your joints". Stretching your joints is a bad idea because joint laxity produces instability and weakness.

All you really need is the lengthening of certain muscles. There are only a few muscles involved in most men's loss of range of motion. This is key.

There are 2 simple stretches everyone needs. You can do them in only minutes a day, and once every other day once you regain your flexibility.

Flexibility is a Sign of Youth

Losing flexibility as we age is the rule. You accelerate the loss if you sit all day. Proper stretching can slow the decline dramatically. Maintaining youthful flexibility can ward off the aches and pains associated with aging and inactivity.

Before you stretch, you should understand this important distinction: Tendons attach your muscles to your bones while ligaments attach bones to bones. Healthy stretching helps lengthen muscles and strengthens tendons but shouldn't put pressure on ligaments.

Contrary to popular belief, you don't want loose joints. The tighter they are, the more stable and stronger they are. The stronger they are, the less likely they are to suffer injury and the less pain you will feel. What you want is long and relaxed muscles that can lengthen without resistance on demand. This is critical in a couple of key muscle groups.

Before you start a stretching program, I need to point out one more distinction. Passive stretching does nothing to warm you up. Use these stretches after activity or exercise – not as a warm-up.

I agree with my colleague Bob Arnot, M.D. who said "Stretches make a poor warm-up. Studies have shown that they create more injuries than they prevent when muscles are cold and stiff. A muscle shouldn't be stretched until it's warm and pliable."

Two Stretches in Two Minutes

You don't need marathon stretching sessions. My *2 stretches, 2 minutes* program will help you maintain natural flexibility for life.

The two parts of your body that you should stretch daily are the front of your shoulders and the front of your hips.

➤ **Shoulder Stretch** - You need to stretch these muscles because they shorten from most types of work. Weight lifting will cause further shortening of the muscles on the front of the shoulder joint. Calisthenics are much more effective in strengthening ligaments and tendons. There is also a lower risk of injury with calisthenics than there is with weight training.

How To: Stand in an open doorway. Raising your arm to a 90-degree angle with palm facing out, press your hand and shoulder against the wall and doorjamb. You should feel the wall against the inner part of your elbow. Slowly, increase the tension as you push forward. Hold for a 10 count. Then repeat with the other arm.

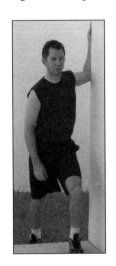

➢ **Hip Flexors** - You need to do this stretch because sitting causes shortening of the muscles of the front of the hip, particularly if you sit for long periods (and who doesn't?) Ninety percent of American adults experience lower back pain at some point in their life. Stretching your hip flexors muscles several times a week will help prevent this lower back pain.

How To: Stand in a modified runner stance, with right foot forward and left foot back, feet flat on floor. Put your hands on your hips and keep your back and hips in straight alignment. Push forward with your hips, while maintaining your erect posture. Slowly, push your hips forward only until you feel a comfortable level of tension. Hold for a 10 count. Switch sides by reversing your leg stance and repeat.

Some sports require additional stretching. For example, if you enjoy kayaking or rowing, you need to stretch your deltoid (back) muscles. Another example would be running or martial arts where it would be helpful to stretch your hamstrings and quadriceps (thighs).

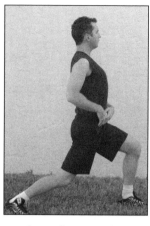

A good source for technique and sport-specific stretches with photos is: *Relax Into Stretch: Instant Flexibility Through Mastering Tension* by Pavel Tsatsouline. It is available through Amazon.com.

Stretching Tips for Injury Prevention

✓ Don't hurry! You should be in a relaxed state of mind before stretching.

✓ Warm up your shoulders by doing circles with your arms before stretching.

✓ Walk around the block before stretching your hip flexors.

✓ Stretch your shoulders and hip flexors after your warm-up and after exercise.

✓ Wait the tension out; don't force it.

✓ Don't bounce; hold the stretch for a 10 count.

✓ You should feel tension, but no pain

✓ Don't stretch through pain; stop! And modify how far you push the muscle.

Secret #5

Beat this Man's Disease

Protect Your Prostate

Every man has a hidden health problem waiting to happen. If you are over 40, yours may have already begun.

The problem involves a dangerous little saboteur that lies between your bladder and your penis – a place where you don't want problems. I'm talking, of course, about the prostate gland – the potential cause of disturbed sleep, incontinence, impotence, disease and even death.

The earliest sign of trouble – *nocturia* – begins as a nagging ache that nudges you from your dreams. You look at the clock (3 a.m.), roll over and cross your legs. It's no use. Pressure turns to pain. And you make another trip to the bathroom wondering whether you'll be able to get back to sleep.

Most of my patients tell me that they don't mind waking up once. Even twice. But when you have to get up three or more times, it's ridiculous.

What's more ridiculous is how common a problem it is. Benign prostatic hyperplasia (swollen prostate) is the number one diagnosis made in American men over the age of 55. And the longer you live, the greater your chances of being afflicted. Eighty percent of American men will get it at some point. If you make it to 80, your probability reaches 90%.

Where Does the Problem Come From?

Such prevalence begs for an explanation. Are we men born with a design flaw? Or… is it something we're doing?

I'll give you the answer to those questions and tell you how to eliminate your prostate problems. But you must begin with an open mind. Because I'm about to show you that most of what you've been told about prostate problems – from the medical mainstream – is seriously flawed.

The flaws begin with a mistaken notion of the cause. <u>This condition is not caused by natural testosterone</u>. Quite to the contrary, it is caused by unnatural environmental pollutants that overwhelm testosterone metabolism.

And guess what? When you have a flawed understanding of causation, you get flawed treatments. Current mainstream treatment strategies for the prostate are flawed.

The typical solutions are cutting (surgery), burning (radiation) and poison (drugs). They do not address the cause and they are fraught with complications and side effects. (See table below.)

RISKS ASSOCIATED WITH PROSTATECTOMY, RADIATION AND CHEMICAL CASTRATION

	Prostatectomy	Radiation	Chemical Castration
Impotence	30 - 60%	40 - 60%	5.4%
Incontinence	5 - 15%	< 1%	14.9%
Heart Attack	.4%	N/A	12.5%
Death	.1 - 2%	< 1%	N/A
Urethral Obstruction	.6 - 25%	4%	N/A

(Adapted from Catalona, William J., M.D. in Fox, Arnold, M.D. and Fox, Barry, Ph.D., The Healthy Prostate, 1996, John Wiley and Sons, Inc., NY, NY. pp. 219.)

The alternative treatments I've seen also show an inadequate understanding of the cause. Although they are much safer than mainstream interventions, they are equally ineffective.

The real cause comes from the environment. We are doing things to tell our prostates to grow. The prostate is doing nothing but following orders – commands given at the cellular level by an environmental deluge of hormonal pollutants – DHT, estradiol and a host of mimickers.

The Choice is Yours: Keep Your Prostate Healthy

When you understand the cause, you can change it. When you change the commands – it will stop growing. You can have a trouble free prostate no matter how long you live.

I've seen hundreds of men do it naturally – without surgery and without drugs. And I've seen the results. No more nocturia. No more leaking urine. No more burning with urination. No more sexual dysfunction. No more pain.

The Rule of the Hammer

The hormonal understanding of the cause of prostatic enlargement appears to have escaped urologists. After all, they are surgeons. There is an axiom in psychology called "The Rule of the Instrument".

I call it the rule of the hammer because my 4-year-old son, Dylan illustrates it perfectly. If I give him a toy hammer, everything in the house needs hammering.

In other words, we think of using the tools we know first. Surgeons know surgery. They have been put in charge of prostate health in this country. The result is 400,000 surgeries on the prostate per year.

My experience has taught me to put my faith in nature and search for something unnatural that we were doing wrong. That search has led me to conclude that we have taken a perfectly designed prostate and created a monster with unnatural hormonal pollutants. Of course, our prostates will swell if we constantly give them the hormonal signals to grow!

Your prostate is the male equivalent of the uterus in women. They both originate from the same group of cells in development. Like the uterus, your prostate is hormonally derived and hormonally controlled.

Give your prostate a daily bath of the powerful growth stimulating hormones dihydrotestosterone (DHT), estradiol and estrone and you transform mild mannered David Banner into the raging Hulk. The problem with this transformation is that The Hulk doesn't fit in Dr. Banner's clothes.

Tracking Down the Real Cause

It started in the early 90's when studies appeared showing lower than average testosterone levels in men with both benign enlargement of the prostate and prostatic cancer. This blew the conventional wisdom that prostate disease was caused by testosterone out of the water.

Since testosterone is the hormone that makes a man a man, this mistaken notion of the cause had led doctors to believe it was an inevitable consequence of being a man. Now that this theory is disproved, there is hope that a man can beat prostate disease without giving up his manhood.

I was first put on the trail of an environmental cause at about the same time when population studies began showing a bulk of evidence that prostatic disease is a curse of industrialized nations. It is rare in third world countries, very common in developed countries and rising rapidly in emerging countries.

But one study really stood out. In 1993, a European report revealed that prostatic disease rates in American blacks were the highest of any group on earth. But rates for the same diseases in African blacks were among the lowest.[1]

Another group with very low rates of prostatic problems is Asian men with the Chinese fairing the best. But if that Chinese man moves to American? You guessed it. His risk rapidly catches up to the average American born man. In other words, for African-Americans and Asian-Americans, living in the US is a bigger risk factor for prostatic disease than genetic make-up.

Another clue came from the study of men born with a rare deficiency of the enzyme 5-alpha-reductase. It converts testosterone to dihydrotestosterone (DHT). Men without it have very low levels of DHT but normal or high testosterones. Prostatic disease in this group is extremely low.

Ask Your Doctor to Measure DHT

Subsequent studies have found DHT to be much more powerful than testosterone at stimulating prostate growth. It binds to growth receptors on prostatic cells. When DHT binds to these receptors it signals the prostatic cells to grow and proliferate. It is concentrated in prostatic tissue and even higher in diseased prostates. And while testosterone declines with age, concentrations of DHT in the prostate increase with age.

DHT can now be measured in your blood. It's not routinely done but your doctor can order it if you ask. I have found it to be quite valuable. In my patients who have a DHT in the upper half of normal, I usually recommend that they take action to lower it. Why would I urge action when DHT is "normal"? To answer that I have to explain what your laboratory means by "normal"

It's not complicated. The "normal value," sometimes called "reference range" is the middle 95% of the population. Since 80% of American men will get enlargement of the prostate and DHT is the most powerful stimulator of prostatic growth, a "normal" DHT might not be that desirable.

Keep Your DHT Low the *Natural* Way

The role of DHT in enlargement of the prostate has not escaped the attention of the pharmaceutical industry. The prescription drug finasteride (Proscar) works by inhibiting the production of DHT. It works reasonably well and I prefer it to the other prescription medications available. Side effects, however, including decreased libido, enlarged breasts and impotence, can be a problem with Proscar. And non-prescription alternatives work equally well without the side effects.

The common herb saw palmetto has also been shown to inhibit the production of DHT. In fact, a 1996 study in *Prostate* compared the effectiveness of saw palmetto and Proscar and found them to be equal.[2] But I've never seen a single case of impotence (or any other serious side effect for that matter) from saw palmetto.

Another study of Saw Palmetto showed that it is the most effective among phytonutrients for relieving the symptoms of BPH.[3]

Even the normally anti-herb, anti-supplement, anti-nutritional remedy publication JAMA (Journal of the American Medical Association) made a rare concession over saw palmetto. In November of 1998, after reviewing the evidence from multiple scientific studies, the report concluded, "extracts from the saw palmetto plant, *S. repens*, improve urinary tract symptoms and flow measures in men with BPH."

Other researchers have found that saw palmetto extract inhibits up to 90% of the conversion of testosterone to DHT. This is astounding to me. The Native Americans that handed down the tradition of using saw palmetto could not have known about DHT. Yet they used it in men with urinary flow problems.

Plant products used as traditional medicines in other parts of the world have also been found to inhibit DHT. I have long recommended and used extracts of pumpkin seed, Pygeum bark and stinging nettle. It turns out they all have one thing in common with saw palmetto. They contain a powerful DHT blocker called beta-sitosterol.

Beta-Sitosterol: Nature's Prostate Protector

New research shows beta-sitosterol to be the main active ingredient in each of these traditional remedies. Beta-sitosterol has been extracted from these plant sources and subjected to studies on BPH. One randomized, double-blind, placebo controlled study performed by Ruhr-University in Germany, tested the effectiveness of beta-sitosterol on BPH symptoms. The study concluded that beta-sitosterol improved urinary flow and overall symptoms of BPH.[4]

Another study in Great Britain[5] and another in Japan[6] reported similar findings.

I have used it in my practice to good effect and have seen or heard no reported side effects. In Europe, it is sold by prescription only. In the US, it is available as a nutritional supplement. The studies I've seen proving effectiveness used doses from 40 mg to 200 mg per day.

So the trumped up testosterone derivative DHT is the principle engine driving the enlargements of the prostate. And DHT can be blocked by natural plant derivatives like saw palmetto extract and beta-sitosterol. But why are DHT levels in the prostate higher in older men while testosterone is declining? And why is prostate disease such a sure bet in older men living in industrialized nations? The answer reads like 1950's science fiction.

The Plague of the Modern World

The reason prostates grow in industrialized nations can be summarized with one word – *xenoestrogens*. Produced by the millions of tons, they are set loose on nature by modern industry. In biology, "*xeno*" means foreign or alien.

In Secret #2, I talked about the feminizing effect of chemicals in the environment. Alien estrogens are the other side of that same coin.

About fifty years ago, modern industry started to release these chemicals into the environment in massive quantities. Years later, peculiar hormonal abnormalities began to show up.

Here's another shocking story about the effects of estrogens in your environment. This one comes from a research team at Tufts University in Boston.[7]

The researchers uncovered link after link between environmental chemicals and hormonal effects in both wildlife and humans. "*Aviation crop dusters handling DDT were found to have reduced sperm counts.*" Factory workers producing other insecticides, *"lost their libido, became impotent and had low sperm counts."*

"Man-made compounds used in the manufacture of plastics were accidentally found to be estrogenic... For example, polystyrene tubes released nonylphenol, and polycarbonate flasks released bisphenol-A... Bisphenol-A was found to contaminate the contents of canned foods; these tin cans are lined with lacquers such as polycarbonate. Bisphenol-A is also used in dental sealants and composites. We found that this estrogen leaches from treated teeth into saliva: up to 950 micrograms of bishenol-A were retrieved from saliva collected during the first hour after polymerization."

"Other xenoestrogens recently identified among chemicals used in large volumes are the plastizicers benzylbutylphthalate, dibutylphthalate, the antioxidant butylhydroxyanisole, the rubber additive p-phenylphenol and the disinfectant o-phenylphenol. These compounds act cumulatively. In fact, feminized male fish were found near sewage outlets in several rivers in the U.K.; a mixture of chemicals including alkyl phenols resulting from the degradation of detergents during sewage treatment seemed to be the causal agent."

The report goes on... page after page of hormonal mutations linked to industrial pollutants.

This barrage of xenoestrogens is overwhelming to a man's testosterone metabolism. Testosterone is depleted and estrogens accumulate.

Many studies around the world have now linked this imbalance of testosterone and estrogen to prostatic disease. A study from Germany published in the *Journal of Clinical Endocrinology and Metabolism* found estrogen levels in prostatic tissue increase in aging men in modernized countries. And they are even higher in men with BPH.

Even more incriminating, a Japanese team researching the problem recently discovered that prostate size directly correlates with the ratio of estradiol to free testosterone. They reported "patients with large prostates have more estrogen dominate environments" and "estrogens are key hormones for the induction and development of BPH."

All Men May Not Need Yearly PSA Test

A recent study concluded that it might not be necessary for every man's PSA levels to be monitored annually. The Health Science Center at the University of Colorado looked at data collected by the National Cancer Institute. PSA levels of around 28,000 men between the ages of 55 and 74 were studied. The study showed that for men with low PSA levels in initial screenings, annual screenings might not be required to monitor their health adequately.

Aware: Newsletter of the National Prostate Cancer Coalition

Enough on the evils of environmental estrogens. What can be done about it? Well, I can't change the entire industrialized world. But I can't help to protect my patients (and maybe you too) from a world gone awry. And we can get help from an seemingly unlikely source.

Lessons from a Bodybuilder

Remember: estrogens accumulate when normal testosterone metabolism is overwhelmed. Well, professional body builders have been intentionally doing this for decades. (I have patients who are third generation body builders.)

They routinely inject themselves with huge doses of testosterone and other androgens to achieve superhuman strength and massive muscles. That's how they make their living. And in the process, they have learned a few things.

One thing all experienced body builders know is this: If they inject high doses of testosterone, they will overload the body's capacity to process it causing an accumulation of estrogen. This results in feminizing symptoms like breast enlargement - the last thing they want.

So they have, over the years learned ways to prevent the accumulation of estrogens. Treating these patients is part of my specialized practice of men's health improvement. And in the process, I've learned a few things too.

Save Your Manhood and Lower Your Estrogen

Like DHT, estrogens can be measured in your blood. And like DHT, there are prescription drugs that can lower estrogens. The drugs are used mainly in the treatment of cancers in women and tend to be heavy handed and toxic. They are replete with side effects especially sexual dysfunction. But again, natural alternatives work as well without the side effects.

Body builders and athletes have used a nutrient called indole-3-carbinol (see Secret #1) to lower estrogen for years. It is naturally found in cruciferous vegetables like Brussels sprouts. Recent research has been proving them right.

A 1997 study appearing in the Journal of the National Cancer Institute measuring urine levels showed significantly lowered estrogen levels in patients treated with indole-3-carbimol.[8]

Another study from researchers in New York and reported in the Journal of Nutrition in December 2000 found indole-3-carbimol to be a potent "down regulator" of estrogen activity.[9]

I3C is available as a nutritional supplement. So in addition to eating your vegetables that contain I3C, like Brussels sprouts, cauliflower, broccoli, cabbage and mustard, you can get extra protection by taking a I3C supplement.

As you know, DIM is another similar nutrient I use when estrogen levels are resistant to treatment. Think of it as a trumped up I3C. Athletes have been using it to good effect and a recent study using rats proved that DIM effectively inhibited estrogen activity.[10]

Even more exciting, doctors at UC Berkeley looked at the affect of DIM on prostate cancer cells. DIM slowed cancer cell growth by 70%. Now that's powerful protection.[11]

Take Action Today

Go back to Secrets #1 and #2. Follow my recommendations for lowering estrogen – including DIM and I3C.

These supplements are easily available and work like a charm.

Secret #6

Stay Virile to 100

Keep Your Passion for Life – Even as You Hit Triple

On the surface, you can observe aging as your hair turns gray, your waistline grows, and your body goes soft. But there are bio-chemical changes underneath, that drive this physical aging. Manipulate what happens at the cellular level, and you can control the way you age. You'll find it's easy to stay younger longer.

You've already seen the importance of testosterone in a man's body. Keeping testosterone up and estrogen down is one of the keys to longevity.

For Secret #6, I'm going to show you the other critical "bio-markers" of aging. I'll show you how to test for, and then reverse these signposts of the aging process.

Most doctors don't pay much attention to these markers. As you'll discover, this is a BIG mistake if you want to hold onto your youth.

In this secret, you'll learn how to take control of:

• **GH** - Nature's Truest Fountain of Youth.

• **Insulin** - The Over-Looked Secret to High Energy and a Lean Body.

• **Triglycerides** – More Important Than Cholesterol for Heart Health.

• **HDL** – The Good Cholesterol No Drug Can Give You.

• **CoQ10** – The Often-Deficient Anti-Aging Nutrient.

• **Body Fat** – The Less You Have, The Longer You Live.

• **Bone Density** – Keep Your Mobility By Fortifying Your Bones.

• **Lung Capacity** – The Little-Known Secret for A Long, Disease-Free Life.

• **Heart Capacity** – One of the Central Keys to Longevity.

Each of these nine points undergoes a transformation as you age. Taking control of them starts with getting a blood test to check your levels and then using specific anti-aging therapies to improve them. Others require exercise and a proper diet.

Let's start with one of the most promising anti-aging discoveries ever…

Human Growth Hormone: Your Most Powerful Anti-Aging Secret

Human growth hormone or GH is the closest thing to the Fountain of Youth we have. Your body produces high amounts of GH when you're young, but production declines throughout your adult life. GH is responsible for rejuvenating and repairing all tissues in your body. As your GH declines, it orchestrates many of the changes of aging. Changes like loss of muscle tone, wrinkles, energy decline and excess fat gain. But *add* GH back, and you reverse some of these consequences of aging.

A recent study at the National Institutes on Aging once again proved that GH improves lean body mass and decreases body fat – even in healthy men.[1] Studies also show it improves strength, sexual capacity, physical function and reduces frailty in elders.

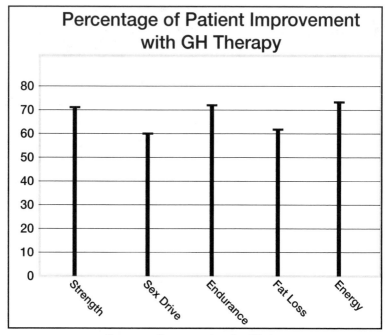

Source: Cenegenics Institute

So how do you use GH? I've found you can elevate GH in three ways:

1. **Eat More Protein**: Since GH helps you build muscle, and when you eat high amounts of protein you have the material to build muscle, it makes sense that your GH would rise in response to a high protein diet. And indeed, it does. This is a mild elevation, but nonetheless, GH is so powerfully beneficial, even a slight increase can make a big difference.

2. **Perform Strenuous Exercises**: Strenuous exercise also increases levels of GH in your body. Now I'm not talking about a brisk walk around the block; I mean gut-wrenching exercises like

heavy squats and dead lifts. This is not a tip for the faint of heart. But if you're athletic and in good shape, you should try it.

3. **GH Injections**: If you want real GH, it must be by injection and a doctor must prescribe it. You must get your blood levels of GH checked. If your doctor will authorize it, you can get a handy GH cartridge for home use without needles. I've used it in patients from 35 to 95 years old at my Wellness Center in south Florida. I've seen some remarkable changes with GH.

High Levels of Insulin: Your Number One Risk for Obesity

When you hear the word "insulin," you think of diabetes. But insulin isn't just about this disease. Even if you aren't diabetic, you can still benefit from having your insulin levels measured. Why? Because insulin plays a key role in aging.

Insulin tells your body to build fat. The more insulin you have, the more fat you'll pack on. Most hormones decline with age, but insulin increases with age. If you want to stay lean, strong and vigorous at any age, keep your insulin low.

Optimize Your Insulin	
Risky	20 and up
Normal	11 to 20
Best Anti-Aging	3 to 10

To control insulin it's very important you maintain your blood sugar with a low carb diet. Remember, focus on protein and avoid processed foods. Use the Glycemic Index on my website as a guide to help you choose the healthiest carbs. And remember to exercise.

What's More Important than Cholesterol for Avoiding Heart Disease?

Triglycerides are a type of fat in your blood. High levels put you at risk of heart disease. What's more, as you age, your triglycerides can rise. That's why it's essential to get a triglyceride test. Here's an idea of where yours should be if you want to maintain a healthy heart:[2]

The Truth About Your Triglycerides	
High	200 mg/dl or higher
Risky	150 to 199 mg/dl
Best Anti-Aging	Less than 100 mg/dl

The most effective way to lower triglycerides is to make the focal point of your diet lean protein. Protein from fish and grass-fed beef is best because these animals have healthy levels of omega-3s. These good fatty acids will also help to reduce your triglycerides, not to mention your waistline.

HDL: The "Good" Cholesterol

HDL is the good kind of cholesterol. HDL delivers life-giving nutrients and helps remove the bad LDL cholesterol from your arteries. Although a certain amount of LDL in your blood is normal and healthy, excess LDL often accumulates in elders. When this happens, doctors often prescribe cholesterol-lowering drugs.

But if your doctor tries to put you on cholesterol medication, be warned. Those drugs lower LDL, but they don't increase HDL – and that's what matters. Whether you have high cholesterol or not you should work to increase your HDL to above 80…

The Truth About Your HDL	
	HDL
Risky	40 or below
Normal	Above 40
Best Anti-Aging	Above 80

Boost Your CoQ10 and Increase Your Lifespan

CoQ10 plays a key role in creating the energy you use to function. It's an anti-oxidant and can help prevent and even *reverse* heart disease. CoQ10 can improve your immune system, reverse gum disease and increase your overall energy.

Unfortunately, once again, CoQ10 levels decline with age, as much as 80% through the years. Studies link this decline to the diseases and illnesses of aging, especially cardiovascular problems.[3] In fact, most of my heart patients have turned out to be deficient in CoQ10.

You can measure this critical nutrient in your blood but very few doctors order it. You will have to ask. It's imperative you get your levels checked and see how much CoQ10 anti-aging power you're missing. Then you can start doing something about it. First, you can add more CoQ10 to your diet by eating red meat and eggs. However, modern animal husbandry has led to lower levels of this anti-aging wonder so supplementation is important. For maximal anti-aging benefit, I recommend taking between 150 to 300 mg per day.

A Growing Waistline Accelerates the Aging Process

Increasing body fat is a *physical* marker of aging. If you don't act to prevent it, fat slowly but relentlessly moves into your cells and pads your waist for no reason other than age. Again, this shift is not inevitable. You can manage it if you know how.

In Secret #4, you learned that muscle mass is critical for living a strong, healthy life – and retaining your mobility far into old age. Fat is the flip-side of this coin.

Several tests can identify and track this change in fat. The most accurate test is the hydrostatic body fat test. It works like this: you get into a tank of water and go under.

Test takers record your weight while you're underwater. You can get a hydrostatic test at some health clubs, university health centers and hospitals. You can also measure fat yourself with a set of calipers. What's a youthful body fat range for a man? 10-14%.

Do you need to drop a few pounds of fat? Don't jump on the treadmill just yet. Fat loss starts with adequate protein. *Over-consume protein, and minimize everything else.* This is the one piece of advice where I get the most resistance. If you can have some faith and try it, you'll see too how much easier it makes losing weight and achieving a more youthful body.

Finally, you need to perform *effective* fat burning exercise. Short bursts of exercise burn fat best. Short bursts will use energy from carbohydrates stored in muscle rather than from fat. Carbs are capable of burning energy at a much higher rate. You then burn much more fat for energy during the recovery period as you replenish the carbs. Short bursts of exercise are better for your heart and lungs too.

Build Your Bones for an Age-Resistant Frame

Bone loss is another physical marker of aging. Just like muscle, you lose bone every year. In fact, research shows adults lose 1% of bone mass annually. With loss of bone minerals, your bones become lighter, more porous, weaker and at greater risk for fracture.[4]

Unfortunately, ordinary X-rays can't detect bone loss in its early stages. A bone must lose at least a full quarter of its weight before a standard X-ray can see the problem. Instead, get a bone mineral density test (BMD). The best BMDs test the bones of your lower spine and hip. These areas are at higher risk for fracture as you age.[5]

If your BMD detects trouble, you can increase bone density and strength with weight-bearing exercise such as walking, bicycling, swimming or weight training. Focus on increasing intensity in all of these exercises. Taking calcium will have little effect on this hormone-driven loss of bone with age. You can help reverse the process with the only vitamin that is actually a hormone, vitamin D. For maximal anti-aging preservation of bone, take 400 IU of vitamin D daily.

Maximize Your Lung Capacity for a Disease-Free Life

As the years pass, your lung volume decreases making lung capacity one of the best markers of physical age. As your lung capacity drops, your chance of illness, disease and infection rises. This is why older people are so vulnerable to things like the flu and pneumonia.

Your doctor can give you a pulmonary function test (PFT) to check your lung capacity. This test is not invasive or dangerous. I find it very valuable at my Wellness Center to monitor the benefits of exercise at reversing the loss of lung volume that afflicts so many elders.

I have found that the right physical challenge can reverse this loss of lung volume. For fast results, use a progressive exercise plan like my PACE° program. (See my website for details.) The idea behind PACE° is to advance the intensity of your exercise gradually through time. As simple as this seems, very few people do it. But this is what makes all exercise effective.

Build Your Ageless Heart

Many men don't realize something's wrong with their heart until it's too late. Usually when they're in the emergency room after a heart attack. Yet the real problem started years earlier. You can measure this gradual loss of heart capacity.

You can easily gauge your heart with a resting and recovery heart rate. Let's do resting first. Locate your pulse, anywhere an artery passes close to the skin will do. You can use your wrist, neck, temple, or top of the foot. Most people use the wrist. If you can't feel the pulse in your wrist, place the same two fingers just to the side of your Adam's apple, in the soft hollow area at the side of your neck.

Your pulse should have a steady, regular rhythm. Your heart rate will increase slightly when you deeply inhale and drop slightly when you exhale. Count the number of beats for 15 seconds, then multiply by 4 to get the beats per minute. See how you rank using the chart below.[6]

Check Your Resting Heart Rate	
Fitness level	Beats per minute (BPM)
Normal Adult	60 - 100
Well-conditioned athletes:	40 - 60

How Strong Is Your Heart?

Now check your recovery heart rate. It's a good gauge of heart fitness. To start, walk out and get the mail, or walk around in your house for a couple of minutes. Then take your pulse. Remember the number; it's your normal activity heart rate.

For the next step, begin cardio exercise. Gradually increase the level of intensity in your work effort. Then, at the peak of your intensity measure your heart rate again. Next, decrease your intensity back to normal, check your heart rate until it's the same as it was when you went to get the glass of water. The amount of time from peak activity back to your normal-activity heart rate is your recovery time. The fitter you are, the faster your heart rate will recover back to normal.

If you don't do much short burst cardiovascular exercise, your cardiovascular system probably needs some work. Here's what to do. When you're performing your PACE® short bursts of exercise, try to get your heart rate within the target range for your age. (These ranges use the maximum heart rate of 220 minus your age.) You can start at 60% of your maximum heart rate. After you've worked on PACE® for a few weeks work up to 80% of your maximal heart rate.

Recapture the Strength and Speed of Your Youth

Slowing down and growing weaker are natural parts of the aging process. Twenty-one frail elder subjects recently took part in an 11-week exercise program. After the program, the men showed an improvement in balance, strength, and physical ability, making them less likely to fall.[7]

The old school approach to exercise is still my preference for restoring strength and quickness. Remember calisthenics? They're exercises consisting of simple body movements without weights or equipment. Calisthenics was born out of gymnastics.[8] The word calisthenics comes from the Greek words 'kallos' for beauty and 'thenos' for strength. The purpose is to use your own body for resistance. Here's how to do some of the basic exercises…

Essential Calisthenics for Speed, Strength & Fitness

Half Sit-ups: With your hands on your hips, lift your upper torso off the ground slightly. Your middle/lower back will remain on the floor. Lower gently and repeat.

Push-ups: Start face down on floor, palms against floor under shoulders, toes curled up against floor. Push up with arms keeping a straight line from head through toes. Lower to within a few inches of floor and repeat. This exercise is great for your entire upper body.

Knee bends: Start with your feet shoulder width apart and arms at your side. Lower yourself by bending your knees until your thighs are parallel to the floor, rising up on your toes, while swinging your arms forward until they are parallel to the floor. Reverse this motion and return to your original starting position. Repeat.

Jump squats: Start with your body crouched, feet together, arms at your sides, head straight and level. From this position, quickly straighten your legs and jump upward as high as you can, simultaneously extending your arms and reaching overhead. Once you have landed, return to your original starting position, taking care not to lose your balance throughout the exercise.

Inverted Bicycle: Lie on your back and place your hands under your hips. Lift your legs and begin moving your legs in a cycling movement in the air above your head. Keep your legs moving.

Scissors: Lay on your back. Lift your feet 6 inches off the floor. Open and close both legs about 3 feet apart, keep your legs straight and off the floor. Keep your legs moving.

Get started on your heart and lung empowering exercise program today. You'll have to build up to some of the exercises. Begin nice and easy. Should you feel any pain, dizziness or shortness of breath, slow down. If you'll try them, the age-defying results will surprise you. In just weeks, you'll begin to see a change in your body. You'll feel and look more fit, more energized **and younger!**

Secret #7

Take Your Single Most Important Supplement

Discover the High-Energy Fuel Most Doctors Completely Ignore

When Frederick Crane discovered this bright orange oil in 1953, no one knew its role. By the 1960's Japanese researchers recognized its important role in proper heart function.[1] Since then, over 100 studies have shown its direct link to the prevention of heart disease.

But preventing heart disease is just one of the benefits of this miracle nutrient. It also treats cancer, AIDS, high blood pressure, Alzheimer's Disease and gum disease just to name a few.

The miracle nutrient I'm talking about is Co-enzyme Q10 or CoQ10.

Although you've read a bit about it in the previous secret, it deserves a section all its own. It's that important to your health.

Why You Won't Hear About CoQ10 from Your Doctor

Chances are you won't hear about this super nutrient from your doctors. And if you ask them about it, they'll probably say they've never heard of it. Why? Because most doctors aren't trained in the use of nutrients. And most researchers know it only by its scientific name, ubiquinone.[2]

Although CoQ10 is widely used in Japan, Europe and Israel, it's virtually ignored by the majority of cardiologists and conventional medical doctors in the U.S. for several reasons:[3]

1. Some physicians are dead-set against any natural medicine, including CoQ10.

2. The limited bioavailability of CoQ10 when administered orally has created a myth that you can't absorb CoQ10 and discouraged clinicians. The development of newer hydro soluble version of CoQ10 has opened up a whole new opportunity for research.[4]

3. Since CoQ10 is a nutrient, drug companies can't make any money from it, so they have no incentive to study or market it.

4. Drug companies don't want to you know their statin drugs deplete the body of this vital nutrient—seriously endangering your health.

Drug companies know about the CoQ10-depleting side effect of statin drugs. One company even developed a statin-CoQ10 combination drug to offset the CoQ10 stripped from the body. But they decided to hold the patent without releasing the nutrient/drug combination to the public. Clearly, the companies recognize that their drugs drain the body of CoQ10, and they have done <u>nothing</u> to educate physicians and patients about this very real danger of taking statins. Instead, they downplay this fact in hopes that the news about this side effect does not interfere with drug sales.[5]

Her Doctor Threw Her CoQ10 In The Garbage!

Unfortunately, most doctors don't know enough about the link between statin drugs and CoQ10 to recommend that their patients take supplements. And some aggressively discourage it—regardless of what studies prove.

For instance, a woman who came to my clinic with high blood pressure was able to stop both blood pressure medications she was taking, and now maintains normal blood pressure after we put her on CoQ10 supplements. She also reported feeling "energized" and having a sharper memory.

But when she returned to her cardiologist to tell him the good news, rather than rejoice in her success, he became irate. He told her CoQ10 could not possibly help her blood pressure and threw her CoQ10 in the trash! Incredibly, this is not the only story like this one. And they all reveal a troubling double standard. Most doctors are well informed of the uses and benefits of drugs but uninformed and suspicious of nutritional solutions.

Unfortunately, without the support of pharmaceutical companies, cardiologists and other physicians, it is very difficult to educate the public on the benefits of CoQ10.

In this secret, I'm going to show you how powerful CoQ10 is for stopping heart disease in its tracks (even reversing it)… preventing numerous other diseases… helping you look and feel younger… and super-charging your energy levels — no matter what your age.

Bulletproof Your Heart

CoQ10 is an essential cofactor your body uses to derive energy. You cannot survive without it. It's a powerful anti-oxidant necessary for every cell in your body.[6]

CoQ10 is essential for the normal function of all your major organs. It is especially important to the energy-guzzling organs, like your heart, brain, kidneys, and liver. It provides your body with "high octane" fuel. But this co-enzyme also gives your body five more vital benefits:[7]

1. Destroys free radicals before they can damage your cell membranes.

2. Prevents arteriosclerosis by reducing the accumulation of oxidized fat in your blood vessels.

3. Eases heart disease, high blood pressure, and high cholesterol.

4. Reduces chest pain and improves exercise tolerance in patients with chronic stable angina.

5. Regulates the rhythm of the heart rate.

Most forms of heart disease have one thing in common: low energy production in the mitochondria (the powerhouses) of the cells. This leads to a condition researchers aptly dubbed: "the energy-starved heart."[8]

CoQ10 helps in the chemical reactions required for energy production. This is essential to keep the mitochondria working efficiently. In effect, CoQ10 provides a virtual Fountain of Youth for the cells in your heart and every other cell in your body.

Prevent a Wide Array of Diseases

Like iron that produces rust when exposed to the air, the energy-making process in your cells produces free radicals (by-products that stress the cell). Once damaged by free radicals, the cell tends to malfunction and cause even more stress, sending it into a vicious downward spiral.[9] This "oxidative stress" has been linked to cancer, arteriosclerosis, heart disease, cataracts,[10] arthritis, Alzheimer's and a number of other diseases.

Researchers have found that CoQ10 helps the body neutralize free radicals in the cell. The same way baking soda neutralizes stomach acid. CoQ10 reduces stress on the cells by bolstering the body's antioxidant defenses and cleaning up free radicals before they can damage the cells. In addition, it's been shown that when you increase levels of CoQ10 in your body, levels of other anti-oxidants go up as well, offering further protection to your cells.

Rejuvenate Your Cells and Ignite Your Energy

As you age, your cells start running out of CoQ10, and the mitochondria simply cannot produce enough energy to meet your body's demands. When stockpiles run low, the mitochondria are less efficient and they may produce adenosine diphosphate (ADP), which is a less potent fuel. Over time, running your body on cheap fuel will take its toll, damaging the mitochondria and contributing to a growing sense of fatigue. But when you restock your body with CoQ10, it can operate efficiently.[11] The result: rejuvenated cells and renewed energy.

Percent of CoQ10 Decrease Caused from Aging[12]	
Tissue Affected	**Percent Decrease of CoQ10**
Heart Muscle Wall	72%
Pancreas	83%
Epidermis (skin)	75%
Kidney	45%
Liver	17%
Heart	58%
Adrenal gland	50%

Why You Need CoQ10 Supplements

CoQ10 biosynthesis is a complex process that requires the amino acid tyrosine (derived from proteins) and numerous vitamins and trace minerals. A deficiency in any of these nutrients can impair the body's ability to produce CoQ10.

While CoQ10 is found in some foods, mainly organ meats, most people do not eat these meats. Even if you didn't mind the idea of eating sheep heart, or cow brains, studies show that today's commercially raised livestock have very low levels of CoQ10.[13] Consequently, the average diet provides less than 10 mg per day.[14]

Aging, environmental stress, a diet deficient in specific nutrients, certain cholesterol-lowering and psychotropic drugs, chronic high intensity exercise and other lifestyle factors also reduce the levels of CoQ10 in the body.

So it's not surprising that researchers say many Americans don't have adequate levels the vitamins and minerals needed to process CoQ10 even for limited health much less for optimum health.[15] To make sure you maintain proper levels, you need to supplement your diet.

Boost Your Body's Supply of CoQ10

I recommend taking 100 mg of CoQ10 per day for anyone who is not regularly consuming wild game but is otherwise healthy. If you have high blood pressure, heart disease, high cholesterol, gingivitis, age-related memory loss, chronic fatigue, or are a vegetarian, increase your dose to 200 mg per day.

You can buy CoQ10 in the form of tablets, chewable wafers, or gel caps at many nutrition stores, but you may have to search for the adequate therapeutic doses I recommend. Powdered capsules are not as well absorbed. Gel caps or chewable forms are absorbed better. Because CoQ10 is a fat-soluble nutrient, take it with fat for optimal absorption.

You can take it when you eat dairy, eggs, fish or meat. You can even take it with a teaspoon of olive oil or fish oil. Grass-fed red meat, eggs and cod liver oil make the best fat choices to take with your CoQ10 because they contain CoQ10 naturally.

CoQ10 has no toxicity even at high doses in animals or humans. Any ill effects are minor and rare, usually nothing more than mild nausea. You can minimize this effect by taking CoQ10 with food.

Are There Any Drug Interactions?

If you use cholesterol-lowering drugs, like statins, that reduce the level of CoQ10 in the body, I recommend you supplement with CoQ10.

Beta-blockers, and certain psychotropic drugs like phenothiazine and tricyclic antidepressants also inhibit CoQ10-dependent enzymes, so you should speak to your doctor about supplementation there too.[16]

Patients on Coumadin therapy need to have a blood test checked at regular intervals, and should take CoQ10 only under a physician's supervision.[17]

If you suffer from any serious health condition, you should consult with your physician prior to taking CoQ10. CoQ10 has been shown to be effective in combination with conventional heart drugs. And with the consent of your physician, it may even allow for a reduction in dosage of conventional medicine.

At our Center for Health and Wellness, *more than half the patients who were taking drugs for high blood pressure were able to stop their medication once they began taking CoQ10.*

Your doctor may not tell you – and the drug companies may never admit it – but CoQ10 is nothing short of a miracle heart energizer!

Secret #8

Beat Inflammation

Pain-Free Joints – In as Little as Two Days

Breakthrough treatments can help relieve your pain and get your joints moving freely again in as little as two days. Recent discoveries are emerging from a new understanding of the cause of these problems. These natural treatments are much safer and they can be quite effective.

One of my patients had suffered from pain in the joints of his legs every day for 20 years. He was finding it hard to run his business and it was and getting worse. "Now I'm so stiff in the morning I can hardly get out of bed. My wife has to wait on me while I limp around like an old man."

It had taken a lot for him to admit the pain was getting him down. I told him that the drugs he was taking could never cure his problem. I gave him natural supplements instead.

The Pain and Stiffness Disappeared

Two days later, he came to my front desk and asked to speak with me. Grinning from ear to ear, he shook my hand. "It's unbelievable. I was so used to the constant aching. I woke up this morning and said, 'Hey there's something missing.' Then I realized it was the fire in my hips that was gone... I said good riddance! I let my wife sleep while I went down and got the paper and made breakfast for the first time in years."

He has since referred several other patients with chronic joint pains to my office and now they are pain-free too. He says he tells everyone because, "I can't believe I took all those drugs. Every time I'd see my doctor he would give me a new drug. The damn things bother my stomach. So he'd just give me another drug."

In this secret, I'll tell you about the natural compound and other effective natural treatments for painful joints. I'll show you why it's smarter to try them first before you resort to prescription drugs or worse yet – surgery.

Drugs Can Interfere With Your Healing Process

Conventional approaches have been ineffective because they do not address the underlying cause. They are chemicals designed to mask symptoms. They tell us each new drug is safe when it's introduced. We keep finding out later, that it too, is just as dangerous as the old drug.

Pfizer's anti-inflammatory drug, Celebrex, rapidly became the top selling drug in the country. Now we know there are more dangerous side effects than first claimed.[1]

Steroid drugs indiscriminately turn off all immune responses. That in effect "ties the hands" of your body's own healing system. You may get temporary relief and feel better, but only because they make your body oblivious to the damage being done. I tell my patients taking these drugs is like, "whistling past the grave yard."

Surgeries too, are of dubious value. The two most popular surgeries for arthritis of the knee were performed many thousands of times before there effectiveness was ever tested. Now, two recent studies have found they are, "no more effective than sham surgery."[2]

Understanding what is happening to cause the pain and inflammation is the first step to resolving the problem. We call inflammation of a joint *arthritis*. When the inflammation is long-term and causes degeneration of the cartilage or bone in the joint, it's called *osteoarthritis*. Osteoarthritis can produce pain in the joint by a number of different mechanisms.

Don't Confuse Pain and Inflammation – They're Not the Same

It's time for medicine to stop treating pain and inflammation as if they were the same. Inflammation is not always a bad thing to have. It is the first step in healing. It is your body's emergency response team. Blood vessels dilate. The injured area is bathed in fluid. White blood cells remove debris and fibroblasts lay down a scaffold-like grid for new tissue to be built.

When you take powerful drugs designed to block this mechanism you shut down your natural system for repair. The joint can never heal.

Secondly, pain in the joint doesn't correlate well with inflammation. Some people have a great deal of pain but when we look at X-rays, we see a normal joint without evidence of inflammation. Other people have severely diseased X-rays with little or no pain.[3]

Understanding how pain and inflammation differ is crucial. This allows us to relieve pain but instead of shutting down healing, we can use nutrients and herbs to encourage the response system to do its work better and faster. Nothing else works as well as the healing system you were born with. And in my many years of study, nothing I have learned is of greater value.

The Science Behind Joint Pain

Pain in a joint is a physiological response to damage. Pain receptors are specialized nerve endings. When pain receptors are stimulated, they send a message through the nerve. It travels through the spinal cord to the brain. Perception of pain in the brain then allows you to react. You can stop the offending activity to ease the pain.

But when the damage has already been done, as in an osteoarthritic joint, the pain doesn't stop with cessation of activity. Yet, once again, your body is smarter than you think. This continuation of chronic pain no longer serves a useful function and it may interfere with the healing process.

So, your body is naturally equipped to ease chronic pain. The nervous system reacts to continued pain with an ingeniously designed system of endorphins. Endorphins are naturally produced chemicals that relieve pain and cause a sensation of well being. But, the feeling is only temporary. In a matter of minutes, enzymes in the body break down the endorphins. And, unless the damage causing the painful sensation has been repaired, you will once again experience pain.

This natural system for causing pain, relieving it and allowing it to remind you if the problem hasn't been corrected should not be turned off. It should be used to your advantage. A naturally occurring amino acid, DL Phenylalanine (DLPA), has recently been shown to do exactly that.

DLPA inhibits the enzymes that break down endorphins. When you slow their breakdown, you cause a greater accumulation of endorphins and a more profound pain relief. And with more endorphins in the body for a longer time, the pain relief is longer lasting.

A landmark study of DLPA was reported at the International Narcotic Research Conference. Arthritic patients were treated with DLPA for one month. Of the participants, 75% reported that their chronic pain was completely alleviated.[4]

John Hopkins University School of Medicine studied the effect of DLPA in chronic pain sufferers. They concluded that DLPA supplementation was 85-90% effective in the control and reduction of chronic pain in participants. The authors noted DLPA was as effective as morphine in the relief of pain.[5]

Wipe Out Joint Pain – *Naturally*

If your joints are afflicted with swelling stiffness, you may need to lessen inflammation. But use as natural a solution as possible.

Here are three natural alternatives:

Nettle: An exploratory study, published in *Complimentary Therapies in Medicine* examined nettle's effectiveness for easing joint pain. 18 participants with joint pain took the nettle supplements. 17 out of the 18 participants experienced great relief from their pain. The authors of the study noted that several of the participants even considered themselves cured of their pain. The study concluded that nettle is an inexpensive, safe, and effective way to ease joint pain.[6]

Stinging nettle leaf is highly used in Europe to aid arthritis sufferers. A 1999 German study in the *Journal of Rheumatology* examined how nettle works on arthritis. The researchers found the mechanism in nettle that inhibits arthritic pain. The active ingredient in nettle acts as a switch that turns off the mechanism that causes painful arthritis.[7]

White Willow: *The British Journal of Rheumatology* reported a study that looked at white willow's effect on arthritic pain. Participants with chronic pain were given a placebo or white willow supplement for two moths. Patients had a statistically significant improvement in pain caused by osteoarthritis. The white willow supplement beat out the placebo in every pain measurement taken.[8]

Ginger: *Pharmacology* published a study that looked at the anti-inflammation properties of ginger. Ginger oil was given to rats with induced arthritic knees and paws. Ginger oil was given to the rats by mouth for 26 days. Joint swelling significantly decreased, while joint mobility increased.[9]

By contrast, there is growing evidence, which indicates that anti-inflammatory drugs actually damage joint cartilage. Anti-inflammatory drugs may also affect blood flow in the kidneys. And, they can affect the kidneys' ability to filter.[10]

Corticosteroids are often used to treat inflamed and painful joints. The side effects of these drugs are horrifying. Corticosteroids are a class of the most dangerous drugs produced. Fluid retention, hypertension, loss of muscle mass, osteoporosis, ulcers, thin and fragile skin, convulsions, glaucoma, and tendon rupture are just a few of the many side effect of these drugs.

If you must have an anti-inflammatory, try the two natural alternatives ginger root and nettle leaf first.

Rebuilding Damaged Cartilage

Once you have controlled the pain and swelling, it's time to focus on repairing the damage. A number of supplements can help to rebuild damaged cartilage.

Below, are two effective options:

MSM (methyl sulfonyl methane): is a naturally occurring sulfur compound found in very small amounts in vegetables, fruits, fish and meats. Research indicates that sulfur is required to repair injured cartilage.

I have seen dramatic reductions in arthritic symptoms with MSM. It is our first choice at the wellness center. I use a dose of 1-gram (1000 mg) per day taken with food. A double-blinded study at the UCLA School of Medicine found that arthritic patients who were given MSM for 6 weeks had an 82% reduction in pain. And further MSM seems to reduce the risks of some types of cancers in laboratory animals.[11]

Glucosamine: In a one study published in the *European Journal of Clinical Pharmacology*, glucosamine was examined. 329 patients with osteoarthritic knees were given glucosamine, the medication piroxicam, or a placebo for 90 days. Glucosamine improved joint mobility almost as well as the medication, and significantly better than the placebo.[12]

A double-blinded study of 178 participants tested the efficacy and the safety of glucosamine as compared to ibuprofen. All of the patients had a least one arthritic knee. The participants were split into two groups. One group took a glucosamine supplement, while the other took ibuprofen for a month. Both glucosamine and ibuprofen significantly reduced osteoarthritis symptoms. But, the glucosamine was much better tolerated than the ibuprofen. The authors of the study comment glucosamine is one of the best long-term treatments for osteoarthritis.[13]

Avoid Calcium and Chondroitin Supplements

If you are a man, you have good reason to be concerned over the health of your prostate. You should be aware of an article from *Health Science International* in July 2002. It was titled, "Natural Doesn't Always Mean Harmless: Arthritis Supplement Could Lead to the Spread of Prostate Cancer."

Chondroitin is a basic building block of cartilage. And it is often used as a supplement to promote cartilage health.

Cancer specialist Charles E. Myers Jr. reports that chondroitin can be found in prostatic tumors. He has written several articles linking chondroitin to prostate cancer. He sites studies that show when tissue levels of chondroitin are high; the spread of cancer is greater.

One study followed men who had their prostate glands removed due to cancer. The level of chondroitin sulfate was measured in the tissues around the prostate for 5 years. In the group with low chondroitin levels, the reoccurrence of cancer was low at 14%. What happened if the tissue chondroitin was high? The cancer returned in 47% of those men.[14]

We now know that chondroitin attaches to a protein called versican in the prostate. We have known for some time that versican seems to help prostatic cancer spread.

Another study published in the *Journal of Urology* is also concerning. It found elevated levels of chondroitin in the tissues of not only prostate cancer but also in men with benign swelling of the prostate or BPH.

Now it is important to point this out. None of this proves that taking chondroitin sulfate supplements will give you cancer. It is however, suspicious. And reason enough for me to advise you not to take it.

Choose Your Exercise Wisely

Everyday we hear about the wondrous benefits of exercise. The word "exercise" is used to describe all kinds of physical activity and if we had more of it, we would all get healthy. Doctors and exercise gurus should know better.

Various exercise activities produce widely varying physiological responses in your body. One may induce a desired adaptation while another will have exactly the opposite effect. Which one you need depends on the change you want your body to make.

If you have painful joints, the last thing you need is additional walking or jogging or worse yet, an aerobics class. Years of spending too much time on your feet is likely the cause. More of this activity, no matter how well intentioned, will only perpetuate and aggravate the problem.

You need exercise that helps your body to compensate for this overuse injury.

Tips to Strengthen and Rebuild Your Joints

Once you have given your body the nutrients it needs to repair damaged joints, the right exercise becomes the most effective treatment for arthritis. Here are some principles that will help you use exercise effectively and safely.

1. **If it hurts don't do it**. Pain in a joint is not like a fatigued muscle. You can't "work through it". If an exercise is painful during the activity, stop immediately and avoid that activity in the future.

2. **Stretch but use passive stretching only**. An active stretch uses your own muscles to move the joint like spinning your arms around to stretch your shoulders. That's what I want you to avoid. Your joints don't need the trauma. In a passive stretch you use the floor, a doorway, a rail or another part of your body to stretch a joint while you focus on relaxing the muscles that move that joint.

3. **Lay off the sports**. I'm a big fan of recreational sports but if you have developed pain in your joints, you probably need to give it a rest. There is an axiom in sports training. "You don't play sports to get into shape. You get into shape to play sports".

4. **Use slow and controlled movements**. When you exercise to rehabilitate an overused joint, special care must be taken not to aggravate it. Focusing your attention on the afflicted joints using a deliberate conscious effort will avoid injury.

5. **Begin with low-stress movements**. In the beginning, select an exercise that will get the joint moving with the lowest possible stress on the joint. My favorite for this is swimming. It takes the pressure off the joint and the weightless movement improves blood flow and healing. If you can't swim, just getting in the water and moving the joint will do.

6. **Build muscle**. When I teach Human Anatomy and Physiology, the students all know that muscle provides movement. But they miss the equally important function for muscle of supporting the weight of the body. Your bones were never intended to support your weight alone. Loss of muscle is a common, rarely diagnosed, cause of arthritic joints. You need muscle bulk to surround and stabilize a joint and muscle strength to help with weight bearing. Resistance training can accomplish both. Studies have shown that even elders in their nineties can restore muscle strength and bulk with resistance training. I will devote an entire upcoming issue to this important exercise tool.

Secret #9

Boost Your Brain Power

3 Easy Steps to a Razor-Sharp Mind

You're running out the door and realize you have no idea where your keys are. As you get older, memory lapses can become frustrating, even disabling. How many times has this happened to you?

But when you tell most doctors your memory's failing, they put you through some tests and tell you it's just part of aging. There is some truth to that statement, but it doesn't mean you have to just sit back and take it. You <u>can</u> hold on to a quick and sharp mind as you age.

Secret #9 is all about brain boosting. You'll read about dozens of strategies that can sharpen your thinking and prevent you from losing your memory and concentrating power as you age. You'll discover the No. 1 thing men should do to preserve and promote mental clarity.

You'll also learn:

- How to beat the brain-destroying effects of cortisol.

- Tools you can use to *reverse* cognitive decline.

- The best way to protect yourself from dreaded Alzheimer's Disease.

- The most effective supplements - nurtients **your brain needs**.

How to Fix Your Aging Brain

One of the most exciting recent discoveries about the human brain is its tremendous capacity to adapt. Your brain cannot only repair itself, but it can modify its structure no matter how old you are. If one network of neurons dies, another network takes over by sprouting brand-new connections. New research shows this ability can help your brain stave off age related decline.

In one study, doctors compared the memories of people in their 20s with those in their 70s. Each group looked at 16 words and tried to remember them. The researchers found that with practice the older group performed *just as well* as the younger people.[1]

So how can some elders remain sharp like this while others slip into dementia? The answer has little to do with genes or luck as you've probably heard...

Protect Your Clarity of Mind

Think of your brain as a dynamic, adaptable system. The neurons respond to environmental factors and stimulation. By stimulating your mind, you preserve your memory, and can even restore the clarity you had in your youth.

One of the most promising studies in this area is still going strong. It's The Seattle Longitudinal Study of Adult Intelligence. Since 1956, Dr. K. Warner Schaie has followed more than 5,000 people, examining their cognitive abilities every seven years. His findings are remarkable.

Two-thirds of the people following a "mental education program" showed significant improvement, often returning to pre-decline cognitive performance levels. What's more, they maintained these benefits well beyond seven years.

Regular mental stimulation also offers another plus: It can protect against mind robbing diseases.[2] New research shows that the more you use your brain the lower your risk of Alzheimer's disease. Researchers at Columbia University discovered that people with less than an eighth-grade education had twice the risk of developing Alzheimer's as those with formal education. And if those with lower educational levels worked at mentally un-stimulating jobs, the risk was three times higher.

The more connections, or synapses, you develop between brain cells from the use of your brain, the more resistant you are to the disease.[3]

But you don't have to go back to school to or switch jobs to kick your brain into high gear and create those synapses. All you have to do is use it—even for activities that seem more like "fun" than like learning.

Playtime for Your Brain

You can play crossword puzzles, which are a favorite of mine. Even the simple ones get you thinking about people, places, and things that you wouldn't otherwise. You also can play word and math games.

You can go to the library and check out books with mental exercises or hop on the internet. There are dozens of websites with great, interactive, memory-improving games that feature mnemonics, recognition, and recall tests.

10 Free Brain-boosting Resources

The following resources offer some great games and mental exercises to get your brain into shape.

Books I recommend:
Keep Your Brain Alive: 83 Neurobic Exercises by Lawrence Katz
Aerobics of the Mind Cards: 100 Exercises for a Healthy Brain by Marge Engelman.
Mind Games: The Aging Brain and How to Keep it Healthy by Kathleen Harmeyer.

There's a good chance your local library will have copies of these books, so check there first. If not, you can purchase them in most bookstores and from on-line sources like Amazon.com

Free Websites:
The Memory Gym: www.memorise.org

EasySurf: www.easysurf.us (click on "Memory Game" from the list that appears on the site's home page)

Cognition Lab (memory games by NASA): www.tinyurl.com/2ulzx

PsychTests.com: www.psychtests.com/mindgames

Find engaging word puzzles at:
www.vocabulary.com
www.wordzap.com
www.etymologic.com

There's also a website called Happy Neuron (www.happyneuron.com), which offers training and memory exercises to give your mind a good work out. It's a great site, but it does require a small subscription fee.

A Quiet Mind is a Healthy Mind

When it comes to your brain, relaxation is as vital for maintaining memory and cognitive abilities as mental exercises. You see, if you're wound up all the time, you're actually killing brain cells.

Stress is a leading cause of mental deterioration as you age. Here's why: when you're feeling stressed, your body produces the hormone cortisol. In moderate amounts, cortisol is not that big of a deal. But in larger amounts, it becomes toxic to your brain cells. Over time, too much stress-induced cortisol ruins your brain's "biochemical integrity" causing the mental haziness, forgetfulness, and confusion often associated with aging.

Cortisol threatens your mental health more as you age. Most of the time, anti-aging involves boosting declining hormone levels. Almost all hormone levels fall as you age, but cortisol is one of the very few exceptions. Cortisol actually *rises* as you grow older.

To preserve a youthful mind, you've got to take the opposite approach – actively work to *lower* your cortisol. You can do this simply by reducing your stress level. Set aside a block of time every day, even if it's only a couple of minutes, for practicing and enjoying relaxation. Here are my favorite stress-reducing strategies:

1. Treat yourself to a massage—frequently.

2. Take a few minutes every day to focus on your breathing for the sole purpose of relaxation.

3. Don't hold in your worries: talk them over with someone you feel comfortable with.

4. Take time for yourself everyday.

5. Meditate. You may be skeptical, but meditation is proven to reduce cortisol, so at least give it a try. You'll be surprised by the results.

Don't Rely on Gingko

You've probably heard that the herb *Ginkgo biloba* improves memory and mental focus. You *can* use Ginkgo to sharpen brain functions over short periods, but don't rely on it long term. It just won't keep working.

Gingko dilates blood vessels, increasing blood and oxygen flow to the brain. However, the dilation doesn't last long. Your body will seek to reverse this effect. Eventually it will compensate and reverse the dilation no matter how much ginkgo you take. So, Gingko, like drugs, simply can't get to the root of cognitive problems. Instead, I recommend supplements that give your brain nutrients.

5 Nutrients That Will Feed—and Strengthen—Your Brain

Supplements that address your brain's nutritional needs work naturally and safely to strengthen your mind over time.

Vitamin B_{12} helps create and maintain myelin, the protective coating around neurons. Myelin not only protects neurons from death; it helps to conduct their messages. As vitamin B_{12} levels drop, myelin's effectiveness plummets. What's more, people with B_{12} deficiencies often develop mental disorders and suffer memory loss. **I recommend taking 500 mcg of vitamin B_{12} daily.**

Pregnenolone is the grand precursor hormone that makes all your other tissue-building hormones such as testosterone, DHEA, and progesterone. Studies show it is 100 times more effective for memory enhancement in mice than other precursors. It works in people too. Studies show it enhances mood, mental performance and productivity.[4] **I recommend a dose of 10 mg per day.**

Phosphatidylserine (PS) is naturally concentrated in brain cells and is vital to precise brain functioning. Its job is to house neurotransmitters and regulate their release. PS supplementation can keep them strong and encourage quick thinking. Studies show it can even restore lost cognitive function.[5] **I recommend taking 200 mg of PS a day.**

Acetyl-l-carnitine (ALC) provides a range of brain protection and improves mood and memory by increasing the release of the memory neurotransmitter acetylcholine. It also protects the brain from damage due to poor circulation.[6] It works by keeping the cell energy going despite blood flow. What's more, ALC helps injured nerve cells repair themselves and function normally once again. **I recommend taking 250 mg of ALC daily.**

Like PS, **coenzyme Q10 (CoQ10)** is also naturally present in your body, but most people can still benefit from boosting their levels even further. CoQ10 helps to produce energy every brain cell needs to function. It also protects the cell from negative byproducts of that energy—byproducts like free radicals that are age inducing. **I recommend taking 100 mg of CoQ10 daily.**

Use It or Lose It

Brain anti-aging isn't all about the latest wonder drug, how smart you are, or how much education you have. It's about feeding your mind with the nutrients it needs to stay healthy, and about keeping it stimulated. And that can be as fun as doing crossword puzzles and playing word games, and as simple as reading the newspaper every day. The bottom line is, the more you use it, the less likely you are to lose it.

Secret #10

Get Your Rocks

3 Important Minerals Every Man Needs

Back on the farm where I grew up, men knew their health depended on the quality of the soil. The more nutrients packed in the ground, the more nutrients turned up in the foods growing in it.

But the way commercial farms work today – quicker crop turnover and constant reuse of the same plots of land – has spelled disaster for the mineral content of our soil.

Based on my own research and experience with my patients, men with mineral deficiencies have higher risks for obesity, diabetes, arthritis, accelerated aging, and even cancer.

Adding fuel to the fire, most men don't get the right message when it comes to minerals. In fact, much of the information you'll find is incomplete, or even wrong. So in the end, most men don't bother with mineral supplements.

They opt for a multi-vitamin and call it a day. And that's bad news, because our bodies demand more of certain rocks for long lasting health.

In the story behind Secret #10, I'm going to reveal the 3 minerals many men lack. Minerals that can defend your body against everything from cancer to heart disease, including one you don't hear much about at all.

You'll discover how to:

• Cut your risk of prostate, colon and lung cancer with a mineral.

• Alleviate joint pain *and* protect your mind with a little known mineral. (Chances are this one's not in your multi-vitamin!)

• Ease the symptoms of diabetes or avoid the disease all together using a mineral. In fact, 90% of all Americans consume less than they need of this rock each day, with the fittest men topping the list!

• Prevent coronary artery disease and protect against rheumatoid arthritis with, you guessed it, minerals.

"I Thought a Multi-Vitamin was All I Needed."

I get that from my patients all of the time. It's no wonder, nutritional supplements and even doctors lead you to believe a daily multi-vitamin offers all the minerals a healthy body needs.

Trouble is, this is far from true. For instance, think about the last time you were sick or suffered from some ailment. Chances are your illness and discomfort were the result of a mineral deficiency. Bold words, I know. But it's true.

Legendary, two-time Nobel Prize winning scientist Linus Pauling pointed out that every type of sickness, disease or ailment is traceable to mineral deficiency.[1] And for men, these deficiencies often involve one of three minerals: selenium, chromium or a trace mineral rarely spoken about called boron.

Beat Joint Pain Forever

Boron is nutrition's most forgotten mineral but ironically, it's one of the most important- - especially for men. First of all, this trace mineral can ease your aching joints. Boron stops COX and LOX, the enzymes responsible for creating pain and inflammation in your body. (Remember COX inhibiting drugs like Vioxx? Well, boron inhibits COX naturally, without the side effects.[2])

But boron is more than just a solution to pain. Just like Linus Pauling thought, studies reveal your blood levels of boron show whether or not you'll develop joint pain from arthritis in the first place. Check this out: in areas where boron intake is 1mg or less per day the cases of arthritis are somewhere between 20%-70%

of the population. In places where boron intake is between 3-10mg, arthritis cases drop dramatically to between 0-10%.[3]

Then there's what boron can do for your bones. There are volumes of evidence showing boron is essential to bone health. Boron works like an unstoppable bodyguard, protecting bone stores of vital calcium and magnesium that create and protect your bones for years to come.[4]

Boron even ignites your brainpower. If you're suffering from cloudy thinking, you could be low on boron too. Scientists discovered those deficient in boron didn't perform nearly as well on cognitive tests as those getting as little as 3.25 mg of boron in their diets each day.

For instance, those lacking boron had a decrease in manual dexterity and hand eye coordination, attention span and perception, even short-term and long-term memory. And this was particularly true of older men and women.[5] These studies alone are reason enough to add more boron to your diet, but the good news doesn't end there.

Lower Your Risk of Prostate Cancer by 64%

Boron's most important benefit is to your prostate. As it turns out, boron reduces risk of prostate cancer by more than *half.* Scientists compared the dietary patterns of 76 men with prostate cancer to those of 7, 651 men without it. They found that those consuming the most boron and eating three and a half servings of boron rich fruit per day along with one serving of nuts, reduced incidence of prostate cancer by as much as 64%.[6]

What's more, boron may one day become a common treatment for those that already suffer from the disease. Studies show boron can shrink existing prostate tumors and decrease PSA. In a study published in the *Proceedings of the American Association of Cancer Research*, scientists watched tumors shrink by 25%-38% with boron and PSA drop between 86.4% and 88.6%[7]

Do you need more boron? You bet. Unfortunately, the usual dietary intake is 1 to 2 mg of boron a day for the average adult and normal requirements for men could be as high as 9 mg per day! What's more, I'm willing to bet boron isn't in your multi-vitamin either.

So what should you do? First, try eating more foods rich in boron. These include plums, red grapes, apples, pears and avocadoes, legumes and nuts. I recommend eating trail mix; there you'll get nuts plus dried fruits, which have a higher concentration of boron than fresh ones do anyway.

You can also take a boron supplement. You'll find boron alone or with calcium or magnesium. I recommend taking 3-6 mg a day.

The 3 Most Important Minerals for Men

Boron	Prevents prostate cancer and arthritis, eases swollen joints, boosts brain power, and promotes stronger bones
Selenium	Protects against heart disease, cancers of the lung, colon, liver and prostate. Also prevents arthritis and eases swelling from the disease
Chromium	Protects and treats diabetes by lowering blood sugar and improving insulin sensitivity. Reduces cholesterol and triglycerides, cuts body fat by suppressing appetite and increasing lean muscle

Selenium: Fight Cancer and Slow the Aging Process

Selenium is another important mineral you need more of to keep your body young, strong and healthy. Here's why: selenium is not just a mineral. Like Vitamin C, it's an anti-oxidant powerhouse.

Selenium can slow down the aging process by protecting you from the oxidation of your body's cells and tissues. This is also how it blocks cancer causing free radicals from wreaking havoc on your body. In fact, researchers studying people across the globe found those with low-selenium diets just couldn't fend off deadly cancers. Time and again they suffered cancer of the colon, liver, lung and prostate.[8]

In fact, the connection between selenium deficiency and prostate cancer is so strong it's caught the attention of the National Cancer Institute. They're beginning a 12-year study involving more than 32,000 men to look at the impact of selenium on cancer. I'll keep you posted when the results start coming in.

Selenium deficiency has another risk too. Studies show some people suffering arthritis have low selenium levels as well.[9] But selenium is not only an arthritis preventative, it's a potential treatment. Preliminary research shows selenium can ease the pain and inflammation of arthritis sufferers by stopping the disease where it starts.

You see, arthritis occurs when the body's immune system attacks healthy tissue. Selenium quiets that response by controlling the body's level of free radicals that wage the attack.[10] And there's yet another benefit men can use. Selenium blocks bad (LDL) cholesterol that promotes plaque build-up in coronary arteries and can lead to heart disease.[11]

Getting Your Daily Dose

As you can see, you don't want to be short on selenium. Unfortunately, you're at higher risk for deficiency than your wife or girlfriend because your body requires more. This is mainly because nearly half of the selenium in your body is in the testicles and seminal ducts and is lost in semen.

If you want to fight selenium deficiency and protect against cancer, arthritis and heart disease you should get at least 55 micrograms of selenium a day. It's a small amount, but that doesn't make it easy to achieve.

You see, selenium is one of the only natural cancer fighters you won't find in high amounts in fruits and vegetables. The best way you can get selenium is from organ meats, garlic, fish or nuts. (Just *one single* Brazil nut eaten right out of the shell will provide you with 100 micrograms of selenium. That's more than what you'll find in most selenium supplements!)

Supplements, of course, are another way to get more selenium in your diet. If you take a multi-vitamin there's probably selenium in its formula. If not, you should switch. And if you've had cancer or are at risk for the disease you should add an additional selenium supplement. You can find these at any health store.

Chromium: Protect Against Diabetes While You Build Muscle

Chromium is another mineral you don't hear too much about, but that doesn't mean it's not important. In fact, when it comes to preventing and treating diabetes, chromium is the most important mineral there is.

Chromium maintains proper blood sugar by increasing your sensitivity to insulin—it's like instant protection from diabetes. What's more, if you already suffer from the disease, chromium supplements can improve glucose tolerance and normalize insulin levels naturally.

On the flip side, people low in chromium suffer from chronically high blood sugar, find themselves packing on the pounds and ultimately can fall victim to diabetes. Deficiency is more common than not. An estimated 90% of all Americans consume less than the recommended amount of chromium each and every day. What's more, if you exercise regularly you'll need even larger amounts of chromium than your sedentary neighbors. Active men and athletes excrete more chromium than couch potatoes.[12]

Chromium also does wonders for your cholesterol and triglyceride levels. Studies show supplements can lower cholesterol and triglycerides by nearly 20%. Supplementation can also help you loose weight and build muscle.

Chromium controls your appetite, especially cravings for sweets, and people supplementing with it lost 50% more fat in a three month time period. That coupled with chromium's ability to carry protein where your body needs it most can also help you lose fat while building lean muscle mass.[13]

How Much Chromium Do You Need?

There's no recommended daily allowance for chromium, but I recommend at least 200 micrograms per day for all men.

For diabetics, larger doses can reverse their over secretion of insulin. In my practice, I routinely prescribe 1,500 mcg per day divided into three 500 mcg doses until the patient's serum insulin returns to normal.

Secret #11

Use Herbs for Manhood

Seven Powerful Herbs for Men – The Ones that Really Work

There is much ado about the dangers of herbs lately. Let's set the record straight. First, there is no herb in common use in America today that is anywhere near as dangerous as even the average prescription drug. Secondly, herb interactions with drugs are a concern only because the drugs are both dangerous and extremely over prescribed.

In contrast to patent drugs, herbs have been widely used since before recorded history. Most of the world still uses herbs as their first choice for medicine. Modern scientific studies repeatedly show that they work and are remarkably safe. They can help you gain and maintain energy, strength and health. Yet you may encounter some roadblocks.

- Medical school teaches next to nothing about herbs.

- Most doctors misinterpret their lack of training as a lack of scientific evidence.

- Drug companies have strong-armed the FDA into suppressing their competition from these ancient healers.

- After massive drug industry lobbying, the senate is currently considering a bill to limit your access to herbs with more restrictions and outright bans.

In this chapter, you'll see how to make smart use of the best herbs for a variety of health benefits, in spite of these obstacles. I'll also key you in on their herb-drug interactions to avoid.

Proven Effective over Thousands of Years

Everywhere man has lived, he searched for plants with healing, protecting or enhancing qualities. If fact, written records of herb use dates back to 1600 BC when the Egyptians made a record of about 700 herbal medicines. Hippocrates, the father of western medicine, recorded more than 300 herbal therapies. Later another Greek physician, Dioscorides, wrote "De Materia Medica" detailing 500 herbal remedies. Doctors used it as a medical textbook for one thousand years.[1]

Over time, different cultures have discovered health benefits in a huge array of naturally occurring plants. With their vastly superior safety record and substantial savings over patent drugs, you'd think our government would advocate them, but instead...

Government Interference at Every Turn

The FDA wants to hinder your freedom to buy and use herbs. Over the past year, the FDA has been attempting to rewrite the rules governing your access to natural medicines. The Senate is currently debating the resulting Dietary Supplement Safety Act of 2003.[2]

 The government currently regulates herbs under food manufacturing guidelines (GMPs) as specified by the Dietary Supplement Health and Education Act (DSHEA) of 1993. The new proposal would replace these regulations with the pharmaceutical drug GMPs. The resulting rising costs would shut down many smaller and medium-sized manufacturers of herbal supplements.[3] The result, for you the consumer, will be a much more expensive but smaller selection of available herbs.

Who would benefit from such a law? Well the FDA would get a lot more money for the application and approval process. And, the drug companies would see their toughest competition crushed.

The Road Less Traveled

Medical school taught me very little about using herbs for health. Even though herbs have been our only medicines for centuries and are still the first line of treatment for 80% of our planet,[4] the modern medical establishment considers them alternative therapy.

They were included in a four credit-hour course on alternative medicine. The doctors at my medical school thought taking an herb was about as scientific as a Tarot card reading.

I knew that those same "experts" were dead wrong in their complete neglect of nutrition. If they could be so wrong about nutritional supplements, maybe they were wrong about herbal supplements, too. So, over my first year after internship, I read over 20 books on the use of herbs. I was delighted with what I found.

Let me make something clear – trying a more time-tested and gentler herb before you take a prescription drug does not make you a New Age kook. Herbs are excellent for minor ailments and ongoing health. For many more serious or acute conditions; herbs may help conventional medicine but not replace it.

With over 15 years of practice using herbs, I have found many are both safe and effective. The FDA's interference is political[5] and unnecessary. That said, you do need to be aware of some cautions. Like anything you ingest, educate yourself to avoid improper usage. Use the following tables for general cautions and for specific use of my favorite herbs. I hope you can use them to enhance your health and avoid the more dangerous drugs.

If Using Herbs Heed These Cautions	
Extra ingredients	Read the label and avoid supplements with unneeded ingredients.[6]
Drug interactions	If you take a prescription drug, coordinate your herb with your doctor.
Standards	Standardized extracts use the effective element studied in trials.
Dosing	Just as with prescription drugs, herb dosages are important.
Liver damage	Chaparral, Kava, comfrey and germander may cause liver damage.
Surgery	Stop herbs two weeks before surgery to avoid blood thinning.

Dr Sears's Seven Herbal Superstars

Hawthorn is an effective heart tonic. It keeps your heart rhythm regular and strengthens heart muscle. Hawthorn also helps your heart deal with stress.[7]

Plant Part	Product Form	How Much	How Often	Interactions
Berry	Standardized capsules	240mg	Daily	Advise doctor if also taking heart medications

Garlic helps prevent heart disease, lowers blood pressure and cholesterol and inhibits abnormal blood clots. It also slows the destruction of brain cells and stimulates new neuronal connections.

Plant Part	Product Form	How Much	How Often	Interactions
Bulb	Clove, tablets, oil or powder,	300 mg	With each meal	With gout med Colchicine and blood thinner Coumadin

Gotu Kola improves memory and temporarily boosts alertness. A traditional blood tonic that improves blood circulation.

Plant Part	Product Form	How Much	How Often	Interactions
Leaf	Dried leaves, capsules	500 mg	With each meal	Take no more than 6 weeks; may increase light sensitivity

Black or Green Tea reduces heart disease, buildup of plaque in arteries, detoxifies, free radicals scavenger, protects against formation and growth of cancer.[8] The original anti-aging herb.

Plant Part	Product Form	How Much	How Often	Interactions
Leaf	Tea bags	2 cups	Daily	Mild stimulant. Use caution if combining with other stimulants.

Saw Palmetto limits the multiplication of prostate cells and reduces tissue swelling. It helps with frequent, painful urination and fluid retention.

Plant Part	Product Form	How Much	How Often	Interactions
Berry	Standardized Extract	350 mg	Daily	May lower result of PSA test.

Tribulus terrestris improves sexual potency and function; increases muscle strength; may lower cholesterol and has anti-oxidant properties.[9]

Plant Part	Product Form	How Much	How Often	Interactions
Fruit	Standardized Extract	250 mg	Daily	None. Can together with Viagra.

Milk Thistle can heal liver damage caused by alcohol and drugs. Use with potentially liver damaging medications. More powerful antioxidant than vitamin C or E.

Plant Part	Product Form	How Much	How Often	Interactions
Fruit	Capsules	300 mg	Twice a day	No serious interactions known but advise doctor if also using drugs.

Secret #12

Have Great Sex for Life

Trouble in the Bedroom?

Erectile dysfunction (ED)doesn't have to destroy your relationships.

I'll show you why erectile dysfunction isn't always the nightmare it appears to be. You'll discover the importance of diet, supplementation, and how your overall health affects your sex life.

Secret #12 will give you some new options and a fresh perspective on an issue you may have felt uncomfortable about before. Food, exercise, nutrient supplements and herbs can all have huge impacts.

The Common Problem No One Wants to Talk About

The great Russian playwright Anton Chekov said that man can survive the horrors of illness and war, and all the tortures of the soul. But the most tormenting tragedy of all time is the tragedy of the bedroom.

I know a lot of men who would agree with that. And talking about it, especially to doctors, isn't the easiest thing to do. In fact, ED is the most under-reported condition in the world. Only a small number of men, about 10 percent, talk to a health professional about it.[1]

Here are a few quick facts about ED[2]:

• ED affects more than 30 million men in the United States.

• More than half of all men over 50 have a problem with ED.

• More than 1/3 of all men have a problem—no matter what their age.

• ED is more common in the U.S. than any other country.

• ED is treatable in a majority of cases.

You may think that ED is only an issue when you can't get an erection at all. Actually, if you lose your erection at any time before you have an orgasm, it may indicate that you have a problem. If you have ED, this will happen at least half the time you try.

In some cases, ED is temporary and will go away by itself. Other times, treatment is necessary.

In the past, some doctors may have told you that it's, "all in your mind." Or, "just relax." Today, we know that ED is often a sign that trouble is brewing else where in your body. But don't rule out the mental side: Recent studies show a strong link between ED and depression. We'll talk about that later.

First, it's important for you to know some of the more common causes of ED.

Paging Dr. Killjoy

ED may be a result of health conditions you already have. If you're suffering from heart disease, hypertension, diabetes or depression, ED may be a side effect.

ED can also be a side effect of many prescription medications. There are over 200 prescription medications known to cause problems in the bedroom. These can affect your desire, your stamina, and your performance. Even ordinary drugstore cold medicines can leave you feeling less than a man.

Here are some of the categories to watch for:

- almost all antidepressants
- many blood pressure drugs
- some indigestion drugs
- most sedatives

Before you worry about ED, have a look and see if you're taking any of these medications:

Common Medications That May Cause ED		
Blood Pressure	Norvasc	
	Vasotec	
	Lopressor	
Antidepressant	Zoloft	
	Prozac	
	Buspar	
Antihistamine	Dramamine	
	Benadryl	
Muscle Relaxant	Zantac	
Digestion	Norflex	

Lowering Your Cholesterol May Weaken Your Sex Drive

The worst offenders when it comes to prescription drugs' effects on erectile function are cholesterol-lowering statin drugs. The big drug companies have spent billions of dollars trying to convince you that statin drugs (cholesterol lowering medications) are the answer to all your problems.

Far from it.

Aside from the other, sometimes lethal side-effects of these dangerous drugs, add one more: clinical proof that statin drugs can cause erectile dysfunction.

That's right. We've known for years that statins have this potential.

As far back as 1996, the Australian Adverse Drug Reaction Advisory Committee, (ADRAC) has been reporting cases of ED caused by statins. Most notably by the statin drug Zocor.[3]

Dozens of men took part in one of their studies. Fortunately, when they stopped taking Zocor, most were able to recover. When given Zocor again, however, their ED came back in full force.

In England, the UK Committee on Safety of Medicines, reported a further 170 cases. As in Australia, the men taking Zocor had more problems than all the other statins combined.[4]

If you think about it, the reason is clear. Statins prevent your body from making cholesterol. Cholesterol is essential for the manufacture of testosterone. In fact, all of your hormones depend on cholesterol.

When your body has a hard time making cholesterol, it has a hard time making testosterone. Low testosterone means a weak performance in the bedroom.

The Canary in a Coal Mine

Believe it or not, there may actually be times when ED is actually a blessing in disguise. A large number of clinical studies show that it's often an early indicator of cardiovascular disease.

One major study found that 64 percent of men who had a heart attack had ED before the event. Almost the same percentage had ED before going to the hospital for bypass surgery.[5]

"Erectile dysfunction is often a result of hidden heart problems. It even precedes angina. It can be an early warning system in that respect," said Dr. Andrew McCullough from the New York University School of Medicine.

The connection between ED and heart disease is pretty straightforward: When plaque builds up in your arteries, blood flow decreases. But sexual excitement causes a demand for greater blood flow. Under normal conditions, the inner lining of your blood vessels release nitric oxide, causing the blood vessels to expand. This expansion enables more blood flow, which helps you get an erection.

When your blood vessels harden, as in the case of heart disease, no expansion can take place. And as a result, getting and maintaining an erection becomes difficult.

In many cases, ED is telling you that blood vessels elsewhere in your body aren't expanding as they should. In other words, you're at risk for a heart attack.

The Missing Puzzle Piece: Depression

Obviously, there are a lot of possible physical explanations for ED, so it's not "all in your head" after all. But you can't completely discount the mental aspect: Depression does play a part in erectile dysfunction.

The follow-up to one of the largest studies on male health, The Massachusetts Male Aging Study, uncovered an alarming statistic: ED is 82 percent more likely in men who are depressed.[6]

But treating depression alone is unlikely to help with ED. Treating ED, however, and following a heart-healthy lifestyle, will often ease the symptoms of depression.

Your First Line of Defense

Think back to the times of our ancient ancestors. Do you think cavemen ever had a hard time getting it up? Probably not. Heart disease was unheard of. And with no processed foods, their testosterone levels stayed high. And they had the advantage of eating a high protein, low-carb diet. Protein is essential for the production of sex hormones.

To get the maximum amount of protein, focus on the "big five:" meat, wild fish, eggs, dairy, and nuts.

Red meat: I consider beef to be among the most nutritious foods. The protein is complete and it's a good source of creatine. Creatine makes you stronger and more energetic. Red meat is also the best source of the nutrient CoQ10, which is essential for heart health. And knowing that there's a strong connection between ED and heart disease, it makes sense that CoQ10 also plays an important role in sexual health. I recommend eating grass-fed beef. It has 20 times more of the important omega-3 fatty acids than commercial beef and none of the hormones.

Wild fish: You've probably heard that fish can be a source of mercury and other toxins. However, you can minimize these risks and enjoy the benefit of this rich source of omega-3s by choosing wild Alaskan salmon, mackerel, trout, or sardines. Chose wild over farm-raised and small over large fish. The highest levels of mercury are in swordfish, shark and king mackerel and tuna.

Eggs: Eggs are the perfect food. I eat them every day. Sure, they contain cholesterol. They don't even raise your blood cholesterol. Sure, eggs contain cholesterol. The developing embryo needs it to produced sex hormones—and so do you. But just because they contain it, doesn't mean they'll raise your cholesterol levels. The bottom line: Eggs do not cause heart disease. In fact, there was never any evidence they did.

Egg yolks have all required fat soluble vitamins (A, D, E, and K), iron, and heart healthy omega-3 fat. The whites have all the water-soluble B vitamins and are the source of the highest quality protein on the face of the planet.

Dairy: Dairy is "liquid meat," and full of good protein. Cheese and whole milk are a great source of calcium and vitamin D. Raw, organic milk is best.

Nuts: Nuts are rich in healthy monounsaturated fat. Walnuts and almonds among the most nutritious with omega-3 fatty acids, vitamin E, fiber, potassium, and other minerals. Other good choices are pecans, macadamias, cashews, and brazil nuts. Enjoy them as a snack instead of chips or crackers.

Other factors like excessive drinking and smoking also have a profound effect on both your performance and stamina.

A few drinks will put you in the mood, but too many will make you useless. And smoking? Let's put it this way: the Marlboro Man doesn't see much action these days. A solid erection requires blood vessels that are flexible and able to expand. Smoking will tighten your blood vessels making them too narrow to channel the amount of blood you need for an erection.

Why a Healthy Heart Will Make You a Star in the Bedroom

Following a high protein diet will not only help you in the bedroom, it will keep your heart healthy too. And an explosive new study shows that a healthy heart may be your ticket to a long and satisfying sex life.

Scientists at the University of South Carolina discovered a link between HDL (good) cholesterol and ED. As I've been saying all along, your HDL level is the most important factor in determining your risk for heart disease. Now, that advice is proving to be just as important in the bedroom.

The doctors in South Carolina found that men with an HDL level of 60 mg/dl drastically reduced their chance of having ED. Men with an HDL level of 30 mg/dl, were 66 percent more likely to develop a problem with ED.[7]

L-Arginine: Nature's Hydraulic Pump

Not only does L-arginine improve cholesterol levels, relieve heart-related chest pains (angina), and control blood pressure, it can also help you get an erection.

An erection depends on the expansion of blood vessels. The gas molecule that helps cause this expansion is nitric oxide. Released by the inner lining of your blood vessels, nitric oxide helps to relax smooth muscle tissue and expand the blood vessels in your penis. L-arginine helps create nitric oxide.

Current studies support the use of L-arginine to ensure that the level of nitric oxide is high enough to keep blood flowing to the penis. One study showed an 80 percent improvement in erectile function for men who took 2.8 grams of L-arginine for two weeks.[8]

Another study, which specifically focused on men with ED, showed that more than 1/3 of the men who took 5 grams of L-arginine for five weeks reported a significant improvement.[9]

If you're interested in supplementing with L-arginine, I suggest starting with a loading dose of 5 grams daily for two weeks. Then take 2.5 grams daily for maintenance. Never exceed 10 grams a day.

For best results, combine with a healthy dose (25 mcg) of vitamin B12, and a few of the following herbs. I've had great success with them over the years.

Libido-Pumping Herbs

Tribulus Terrestris: This is my favorite herb for men's health. It's been used in Europe for centuries to boost sex hormone levels and has been clinically proven to restore and improve libido in men. Recommendation: 250 mg of Tribulus Terrestris daily.

Muira Puama: Recent scientific studies confirm the powerful aphrodisiac qualities of this herb. In 1990, men suffering from ED or loss of libido took Muira Puama extract. 62 percent of those with loss of libido reported improvement. More than 50 percent of those with ED reported improvement.[10] Recommendation: 100 mg of Muira Puama extract daily.

Yohimbe: This herb is from the inner bark of a tree, which grows in Africa. At one time, the drug made from yohimbe, *yohimbine* was the only medication approved by the FDA for the treatment of ED. Recommendation: 250 mg of Yohimbine extract daily.

Korean Red Ginseng: This supplement is widely taken to help your body deal with stress. Ginseng also increases stamina and energy. It can even improve your testosterone levels. When you consider it also has a positive effect on blood flow, it's easy to see why ginseng would be valuable to maintain an erection. Recommendation: 250 mg of Korean Red Ginseng daily.

A word of caution: I don't recommend taking herbal supplements continuously over a long period. Use them for four to six weeks and then take a break.

Take Charge of Your Sex Life

Erectile dysfunction is a complex issue, but that doesn't mean you have to sit back and do nothing. In many cases, you can get rid of the problem with a natural solution. Discovering your power as a man is some times as simple as removing what got in the way and restoring a natural balance.

By avoiding certain prescription drugs, pumping up on protein, and following a heart healthy lifestyle, you'll be back in the saddle and enjoying a healthy sex life. If that's not enough, try supplementing with the nutrients and herbs

I mentioned. If you still need more help, there is one additional strategy to try.

That Little Blue Pill

Unlike most prescription medications, Viagra does what it says without significant side effects. I've prescribed it to my patients with great results, although I always put the emphasis on testosterone levels. With that in mind, Viagra can be a good performance enhancer.

In spite of its popularity and obvious benefits, Viagra may not be as helpful for long-term treatment of ED.

There have been studies done to find out how men react to Viagra over one to three years. In one survey, more than half the men stopped taking Viagra after three years because it stopped working.[11]

The same study shows that more than 30 percent of the men had to double their dose to achieve the same effect.

The only warning I offer you is this: Prolonged use of drugs like Viagra can mask symptoms of cardiovascular disease.

Don't use Viagra as a crutch. Get to the root of the problem and try some of the alternatives I mention above. They're much more likely to solve your ED problem for good, and help your overall health at the same time.

Endnotes

Secret #1 — Ride with The King: Testosterone

[1] Hamalainen E, Adlercruetz H, Puska P, Pietinen P. Diet and serum sex hormones in healthy men. J. Steroid Biochem. 1984; 20 (1) : 459-64

[2] Dalessandri KM, Firestone GL, Fitch MD, et al. "Pilot study: effect of 3,3'-diindolylmethane supplements on urinary hormone metabolites in postmenopausal women with a history of early-stage breast cancer." Nutr Cancer 2004; 50(2): 161-67

[3] Kim YS, Milner JA. "Targets for indole-3-carbinol in cancer prevention." J Nutr Biochem 2005; 16(2): 65-73

[4] Ashok BT, Chen Y, Liu X, et al. "Abrogation of estrogen-mediated cellular and biochemical effects by indole-3-carbinol," Nutr Cancer 2004; 41(1-2): 180-87

[5] "FDA White Paper: Health Effects of Androstenedione". March 11, 2004. www.fda.gov/oc/whitepapers/andro.html (accessed 4/30/2004)

[6] "DHEA," Drug Digest. (http://www.drugdigest.org/DD/DVH/HerbsWho/ 0,3923,551934%7CDHEA,00.html), 1/24/2005

[7] Arlt W. "Dehydroepiandrosterone Replacement Therapy," Semin Reprod Med 2004; 22(4): 379-88

[8] Vakina TN, Shutov AM, Shalina SV, et al. "Dehydroepiandrosterone and Sexual Function in Men with Chronic Prostatitis," Urologiia 2003; Jan-Feb (1): 49-52

[9] Reiter WJ, Pycha A, Schatzl G, et al. "Dehydroepiandrosterone in the Treatment of Erectile Dysfunction: a Prospective, Double-Blind, Randomized, Placebo-Controlled Study," Urology 1999; 53(3): 590-95

[10] Villareal DT MD, Holloszy JO MD. "Effect of DHEA on Abdominal Fat and Insulin Action in Elderly Women and Men," JAMA 2004; 292(18): 2243-48

[11] Huppert FA, Van Niekerk JK, Herbert J. "Dehydroepiandrosterone (DHEA) Supplementation for Cognition and Well-Being," Cochrane Database Syst Rev 2000; (2): CD000304

[12] Sahelian, Ray MD. "Tribulus Terrestris: Underrated Roadside Sex Weed," Ray Sahelian MD. (http://www.raysahelian.com/tribulus.html), Viewed: 1/25/2005

[13] Gauthaman K, Ganesan AP, Prasad RN. "Sexual Effects of Puncturevine (Tribulus Terrestris) Extract (Protodioscin): an Evaluation Using a Rat Model," J Altern Complement Med 2003; 9(2): 257-65

[14] Li M, Qu W, Wang Y, et al. "Hypoglycemic Effect of Saponin from Tribulus Terrestris," Zhong Yao Cai 2002; 25(6): 420-22

[15] Riley, AJ. "Yohimbine in the Treatment of Erectile Disorder," Br J Clin Pract 1994; 48(3): 133-6

[16] Ernst E, Pittler MH. "Yohimbine for Erectile Dysfunction: a Systematic Review and Meta-Analysis of Randomized Clinical Trials," J Urol 1998; 159(2): 433-36

[17] Sahelian, Ray MD. "Horny Goat Weed: Will it Make you Horny, too?" Ray Sahelian MD. (http://www.raysahelian.com/hornygoatweed.html)

[18] Liao HJ, Chen XM, Li WG. "Effect of Epimedium Sagittatum on Quality of Life and Cellular Immunity in Patients of Hemodialysis Maintenance," Zhongguo Zhong Xi Yi Jie He Za Zhi 1995; 15(4): 202-4

[19] Xin ZC, Kim EK, Lin CS, et al. "Effects of icariin on cGMP-Specific PDE5 and camp-Specific PDE4 Activities," Zhonghua Yi Xue Za Zhi 2004; 84(2): 142-5

[20] Ang HH, Lee KL, Kiyoshi M. "Eurycoma Longifolia Jack Enhances Sexual Motivation in Middle-Aged Male Mice," J Basic Clin Physiol Pharmacol 2003; 14(3): 301-8

21 Ang HH, Lee KL. "Effect of Eurycoma Longifolia Jack on Libido in Middle-Aged Male Rats," J Basic Clin Physiol Pharmacol 2002; 13(3): 249-54

22 Ang HH, Sim MK. "Eurycoma Longifolia Increases Sexual Motivation in Sexually Naïve Male Rats," Arch Pharm Res 1998; 21(6): 779-81

23 Hamzah S, Yusof A. "The Ergogenic Effects of Eurycoma Longifolia Jack: a Pilot Study," Br J Sports Med 2003; 37: 464-70

24 "Erectile Dysfunction," National Kidney and Urologic Diseases Information Clearinghouse. (http://kidney.niddk.nih.gov/kudiseases/pubs/impotence/)

25 Chen J, Wollman Y, Chernichovsky T, et al. "Effect of oral administration of high-dose nitric oxide donor L-arginine in men with organic erectile dysfunction: results of a double-blind, randomized, placebo-controlled study," BJU Int 1999; 83(3): 269-73

26 Windmueller HG, Spaeth AE. "Source and Fate of Circulating Citrulline," Am J Physiol 1981; 241(6): E473-80

27 Waugh WH, Daeschner VW 3rd, Files BA, et al. "Oral Citrulline as Arginine Precursor May be Beneficial in Sickle Cell Disease: Early Phase Two Results," J Natl Med Assoc 2001; 93(10): 363-71

28 Grossie VB Jr. "Citrulline and Arginine Increase the Growth of the Ward Colon Tumor in Parenterally fed Rats," Nutr Cancer 1996; 26(1): 91-7

29 Pohanka M, Kanovsky P, Bares M, et al. "Pergolide Mesylate Can Improve Sexual Dysfunction in Patients With Parkinson's Disease: the Results of an Open, Prospective, 6-Month Follow-Up," Eur J Neurol 2004; 11(7): 483-8

30 van Deelan RA, Rommers MK, Eerenberg JG, Egberts AC. "Hypersexuality During Use of Levodopa," Ned Tijdschr Geneeskd 2002; 146(44): 2095-8

Secret #2 — Don't Let Them Turn You Into a Woman

[1] Colburn T. Our Stolen Future: Are WE Threatening Our Fertility, Intelligence and Survival? A Scientific Detective Story. Baltimore: Dutton Books, 2000, p. 749.

[2] Montague P. Scientists Pretending. Rachael's Environment and Health Weekly. 377. 1-11. 1994.

[3] Hoffman, R. Estrogen Dominance Syndrome, Conscious Choice, Sept 1999.

[4] Auborn, K., et al. Indole-3-Carbinol Is a Negative Regulator of Estrogen. J Nutr 2003 Jul: 133 (7 Suppl): 2470S-2475S.

Secret #3 — Eat Food Fit for a Man

[1] Cordain L, et al., Plant-animal subsistence ratios and macronutrient energy estimations in worldwide hunter-gatherer diets. Am J Clin Nutr March 2000: 71(3); 682-692

[2] Diamond J The Worst Mistake in the Human Race. Discover Magazine May 1987 p. 65

[3] American Journal of Clinical Nutrition Aug 2000; 72: 466-471

[4] Medicine Science of Sports Exercise July 2000; 32(7); 389-95

[5] Journal of the American Medical Association 1997; 278(18): 1509-1515

[6] Journal of the American College of Nutrition 2000; 19(3): 351-360

[7] Journal of American College of Nutrition 1998; 17: 595-600

[8] Journal of Nutrition 2000; 130: 2889-2896

[9] Swedish Scientists Find Cancer Agent in Staple Foods Reuters News: April 23, 2002

Secret #4 — Make More Manly Muscle

[1] Kamel H. Sarcopenia and aging. Nutr Rev 2003 May; 61(5 Pt 1): 157-167

[2] Fozard J, et al., Epidemiologists try many ways to show that physical activity is good for seniors' health and longevity: review of special issue of the Journal of Aging and Physical Activity: The Evergreen Project. Exp Aging Res 1999; 25: 175-182

[3] Brose A., et al. Creatine supplementatopn enhances isometric strength and body composition improvements following strength exercise training in older adults. J Gerontol A Biol Sci Med Sci 2003 Jan; 58(1): 11-19

[4] Elam R., et al . Effects of arginine and ornithine on strength, lean body mass, and urinary hydroxyproline in adult males. J Sports Med Phys Fitness 1989 Mar; 29(1): 52-56

[5] May P., et al. Reversal of cancer-related wasting using oral supplementation with a combination of beta-hydroxy-beta-methylbutyrate, arginine, and glutamine. Am J Surg 2002 Apr; 183(4): 471-479

Secret #5 — Beat this Man's Disease

[1] Walker AR, et al., Cancer Patterns in Three African Populations Compared With the United States Black Populations. Euro J Cancer Prev 1993 Jul; 2(4): 313-20

[2] Wilt TJ, et al., Phytotherapy for Benign Prostatic Hyperplasia. Public Health Nutr 2000 Dec; 3(4A): 459-72

[3] Wilt TJ, et al., Phytotherapy for Benign Prostatic Hyperplasia. Public Health Nutr 2000 Dec; 3(4A): 459-72

[4] Berges RR, et al., Randomized, placebo-controlled, double-blind clinical trial of beta-sitosterol in patients with benign prostatic hyperplasia. Beta-sitosterol study Group. Lancet 1995 June 17; 345(8964): 1529-32.

[5] Br J urol

[6] Hinyokika Kiyo 1998

[7] Sonnenschein C, Soto AM: J Steroid Biochem Mol Biol 1998 Apr; 65(1-6): 143-50.

[8] Minchnovicz JJ, et al., Changes in Levels of Urinary Estrogen metabolites After Oral Indole-3-Carbimol Treatment in Humans. J Natl Cancer Inst 1997 May 21; 89(10):718-23

[9] Meng Q, Yuan F, Goldberg ID, Rosen EM, Auborn K, Fan S., Indole-3-carbimol is a negative regulator of estrogen receptor-alpha signaling in human tumor cells: J Nutr 2000 Dec; 130(12); 2927-31

[10] McDougal A, et al., Methyl-substituted diindolylmethanes as inhibitors of estrogen -induced growth of T47D cells and mammary tumors in rats. Breast Cancer Res Treat 2001 Mar; 66(2): 147-57

[11] Le H., et al. "Plant-derived 3,3-Diindolylmethane is a strong androgen antagonist in human prostate cancer cells." J Biol Chem 2003 Jun 6; 278(23): 21136-21145

Secret #6 — Stay Virile to 100

[1] Rudman D, Feller AG, Cohn L, Shetty KR, Rudman IW, Draper MW. Effects of human growth hormone on body composition in elderly men. Horm Res. 1991; 36 Suppl 1:73-81. Review.

[2] High Triglycerides.WebMD in collaboration with HealthWise Incorporated, August 2004 http://my.webmd.com/hw/heart_disease/zp3388.asp?lastselectedguid={5FE84E90-BC77-4056-A91C-9531713CA348}

[3] Report of the Expert Committee on the Diagnosis and Classification of Diabetes Mellitus. Diabetes Care 20(7) 1997, 1183*1197.

[4] Frank, Bill. Forever Young: 100 Age-Erasing Techniques, New York, NY: HarperCollins, 2003, p. 94-98.

[5] Bone Mineral Density Test Overview, WebMd in collaboration with Healthwise, Incorporated, August 2004. http://my.webmd.com/hw/osteoporosis/hw3738. asp?lastselectedguid={5FE84E90-BC77-4056-A91C-9531713CA348

[6] Pulse Measurement Test Overview. WebMd in collaboration with Healthwise, Incorporated, August 2004. http://my.webmd.com/hw/heart_disease/hw233473. asp?lastselectedguid={5FE84E90-BC77-4056-A91C-9531713CA348}

[7] LaStayo P., et al. The positive effects of negative work: increased muscle strength and decreased fall risk in a frail elderly population. J Gerontol A Biol Sci Med Sci 2003 May; 58(5): M419-424

[8] History of Calisthenics, July 2004. www.encyclopedia.thefreedictionary.com/ Calisthenics

Secret #7 — Take Your Single Most Important Supplement

[1,2,15] Challam, Jack; Coenzyme Q10: It May Just Be the Miracle of the 1990s; The Nutrition Reporter, 12/4/96

[3,4,14,16,17] Co-enzyme Q10 Notes for Medical Professionals; Nutrimedika; www.nutrimedika.com

[5-7,11,13] Sears Al, MD. The Doctor's Heart Cure. Dragon Door Publishing: Minnesota. 2003

[8-10] How CoQ10 Protects Your Cardiovascular System, Life Extension, April 2000 Are You Absorbing Enough CoQ10?; Life Extension Magazine Special Edition, Winter 2004/2005

Secret #8 — Beat Inflammation

[1] Neergaard, L. Risks of Arthritis Drugs Studied. Associated Pres.s April 2002

[2] New England Journal of Medicine 2002; 347(2): 81-88 and Arthritis Rheum 2002; 46(1): 100-108

[3] Family Practice News, Nov. 2002

[4] Ehrenpreis S. Further Studies on the Analgesic Activity of E-Phenylalanine in Mice and Humans. Proceeding of the International Narcotic Research Club Conference. Persimmon Press 1997 June 11-15

[5] Ostrander S. Super-Memory: The Revolution Carol and Graf Publishers NY: 1991, pp. 238

[6] Randall C. et al., Nettle sting of Urtica dioica for joint pain- an exploratory study of this complementary therapy. Complementary Therapies in Medicine 1999 Sept.; 7(3): 126-131

[7] Klingelhoefer S. et al., Antirheumatic effect of IDS 23, a stinging nettle leaf extract, on in vitro expression of T helper cytokines. Journal of Rheumatology 1999 Dec; 26(12): 2517-22

[8] Mills S. et al., Effect of proprietary herbal medicine on the relief of chronic arthritic pain: A double-blinded study. British Journal of Rheumatology 1996; 35: 874-878

[9] Sharma J. et al., Suppressive effects of eugenol and ginger oil on arthritic rats. Pharmacology 1994 Nov; 49(5): 314-318

[10] Shield M. Anti-inflammatory drugs and their effects on cartilage synthesis and renal function. European Journal of Rheumatology and Inflammation 1993; 13(1): 7-16

[11] MSM: The Multi-Purpose Compound. Life Extension Foundation Magazine September 1999

[12] Forster K. Et al., Longer-term treatment of mild-to-moderate osteoarthritis of the knee with glucosamine sulfate- A randomized, controlled, double-blinded clinical study. European Journal of Clinical Pharmacology 1996; 50(6): 542

[13] Qiu G. et al., Efficacy and safety of glucosamine sulfate versus ibuprofen in patients with knee osteoarthritis. Arzneimittelforschung 1998 May; 48(5): 469-474

[14] Cancer Research 1999 May 15; 59 (10): 2324-8

Secret #9 — Boost Your Brain Power

[1] "The Latest Research on How the Brain Compensates for Age" American Foundation for Aging Research (www.healthandage.com), 8/04.

[2] Schaie KW. "The Seattle Longitudinal Study: A 35 year inquiry of adult intellectual development." Z Gerontol. 1993; 26(3): 129-137.

[3] Kotulak, Ronald. Inside the Brain: Revolutionary Discoveries of How the Mind Works. Kansas City, MO: Andrews McMeel Publishing, 1997.

[4] "Understanding Adrenal Function," Dr. Joseph Mercola's eHealthy News You Can Use (www.mercola.com), 8/27/00

[5] Crook T, et al. "Effects of phosphatidylserine in age-associated memory impairment." Neurology 1991; 4(5): 644-649

[6] Calvani M, et al. "Attenuation by acetyl-l-carnitine of neurological damage and biochemical derangement following brain ischemia and reperfusion." Int J Tissue React 1992; 21(1): 1-6

Secret #10 — Get Your Rocks

[1] O'Shea, Tim; 'Minerals: Trace Elements and Minerals'. Safe Certified Organic Products, January 2005

[2] Hall IH, Rajendran KG, Chen SY; 'Anti-inflammatory activity of amine-carboxyboranes in rodents' Arch Pharm (Weinbeim) 328:39-44, 1995.

[3] Newnham RE 'Essentiality of boron for healthy bones and joints' Environ Health Perspect 102 Suppl 7:83-5, 1994.

[4] Nielsen, FH; 'Studies on the relationship between boron and magnesium which possible affects the formation and maintenance of bones.' Magnes Trace Elem 9:61-9; 1990.

[5] Penland, JG; 'Dietary boron, brain function and cognitive performance', Environ Health Perspect 102 Suppl 7:65-72, 1994.

[6] Zhang Z-F, Winton MI, Rainey C' 'Boron is associated with decreased risk of human prostate cancer' FASEB J, 15:A1089, 2001.

[7] Gallardo-Williams MT, Maronpot RR, King PE; 'Effects of boron supplementation on morphology, PSA levels, and proliferative activity of LNCaP tumors in nude mice' Proc Amer Assoc Cancer Res 43:77, 2002.

[8] Greenwood-Robins, Maggie Ph.D. Foods That Combat Cancer, Avon Books, 2004. p 29- 31

[9] Stone J, Doube A, Dudson D, Wallace J. 'Inadequate calcium, folic acid, vitamin E, zinc, and selenium intake in rheumatoid arthritis patients: Results of a dietary survey.' Semin Arthritis Rheum 1997;27:180-5. and Kose K, Dogan P, Kardas Y, Saraymen R. 'Plasma selenium levels in rheumatoid arthritis.' Biol Trace Elem Res 1996;53:51-6. and Heliovaara M, Knekt P, Aho K, Aaran RK, Alfthan G, Aromaa A; 'Serum antioxidants and risk of rheumatoid arthritis.' Ann Rheum Dis 1994;53:51-3.

[10] Grimble RF. 'Nutritional antioxidants and the modulation of inflammation: Theory and practice.' New Horizons 1994;2:175-85. and Aaseth J, Haugen M, Forre O. 'Rheumatoid arthritis and metal compounds- perspectives on the role of oxygen radical detoxification.' Analyst 1998;123:3- 6.

[11] Ozer NK, Boscoboinik D, Azzi A. 'New roles of low density lipoproteins and vitamin E in the pathogenesis of atherosclerosis.' Biochem Mol Biol Int 1995;35:117-24. and Neve J. 'Selenium as a risk factor for cardiovascular diseases.' J Cardiovasc Risk 1996;3:42-7.

[12] MCarty MF; 'Chromium and other insulin sensitizers may enhance glucagon secretion: implications for hypoglycemia and weight control'; Med Hypotheses, 1996 Jan; 83(1): 29-31.

[13] Anderson, RA; 'Effects of chromium on body composition and weight loss.' Nutri Rev. 1998 Sep; 56-(9): 266-70.

Secret #11 — Use Herbs for Manhood

[1] "A Brief History of Herbs," DreamPharm.com (http://dreampharm.com/garlic/western_herbs.asp), July 30, 2004)

[2] "Bill Summary & Status for the 108th Congress," Thomas: U.S. Congress on the Internet (http://thomas.loc.gov/cgi-bin/bdquery/z?d108:s.00722:), Jul 30 2004

[3] Blumenthal M. "Industry Increasingly Nervous about Drug Orientation of FDA's Proposed GMPs for Dietary Supplements: High Costs Threaten Smaller Companies," HerbalGram: The Journal of the American Botanical Council, 2003; 59: 57-58.

[4] "Alternative Therapies," Health Matters Consumer Guides (http://www.abc.net.au/health/cguides/alternative.htm), July 30, 2004

[5] Dembner, Alice. "Herbal Industry Fending Off FDA," Boston Globe, March 26, 2004

[6] Bergner, Paul. "Herb-drug Interactions," Medical Herbalism: A Journal for the Herbal Practitioner (http://medherb.com/92DRGHRB.HTM), July 30, 2004

[7] Kovach S. Brain Boosters! Boca Raton, FL: American Media Mini-Mags. 2000

[8] Carper J. Stop Aging Now! New York: Harper Perennial. 1996

[9] Hawthorn http://www.mothernature.com/Library

Secret #12 — Have Great Sex for Life

[1] Wylie KR. Management of male sexual problems. Update February 6, 2003.

[2] Gaines KK. Recently approved drugs for erectile dysfunction. Urol Nurs 24(1):46-48, 2004.

[3] Boyd IW. HMG-CoA reductase inhibitore-induced impotence (letter). Ann Pharmacother 1996; 30(10): 1,199

[4] "Reports to the Committee on Safety of Medicines (Yellow Card Scheme) of cases of erectile dysfunction thought to be caused by lipid-lowering drugs." Cited in Rivzi K, et al. "Do lipid lowering drugs cause erectile dysfunction?" Family Practice 2002; 19(1): 95-98

[5] Feldman HA, Goldstein I, et al. "Impotence and its medical correlates: results of the Massachusetts Male Aging Study." J Urol. 1994; 151(1): 54-61

[6] ibid.

[7] Wei M, Macera CA, et al. "Total cholesterol and high density lipoprotein cholesterol as important predictors of erectile dysfunction," Am J Epidemiol 1994; 140(10): 930-937

[8] Zorgniotti, AW, Lizza EF. "Effect of large doses of the nitric oxide precursor, L-arginine, on erectile dysfunction," Int J Impot Res 1994; 6(1): 33-35

[9] Chen J, et al. "Effect of oral administration of high-dose nitric oxide donor L-arginine in men with organic erectile dysfunction: results of a double-blind, randomized, placebo-controlled study," BJU Int 1999; 83(3): 269-273

[10] Sears, Al M.D., The T- Factor, pp. 38-54, 2000

[11] Rosen RC, Fisher W, et al. "The multinational men's attitudes to life events and sexuality (MALES) study." Curr Med Res Opin 2004; 20(5): 607-617